ill-equipped for a life of sex

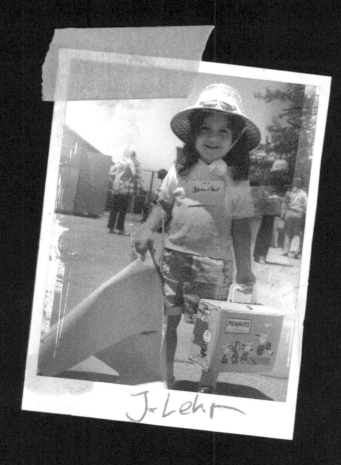

ill-equipped for a life of sex
■ / a memoir / • *by* Jennifer Lehr

1♦ ReganBooks
Celebrating Ten Bestselling Years
An Imprint of HarperCollins*Publishers*

Grateful acknowledgment is made for permission to reprint the following copyrighted material:

Page vii, De Botton, Alain. *How Proust Can Change Your Life.* New York: Vintage Press, 1997. Reprinted courtesy of the author.

Page 36, "Some Enchanted Evening" lyric. Copyright © 1949 by Richard Rodgers and Oscar Hammerstein II. Copyright Renewed, Williamson Music.

Page 95, Red Hot Chili Peppers' lyric reprinted courtesy of Moebetomblame Music, © 1991.

Pages 200–201, excerpts from *Getting the Love You Want: A Guide for Couples (Staying in Love)* by Harville Hendrix. © 1988, 2001 by Harville Hendrix. Reprinted by permission of Henry Holt and Company, LLC.

Page 244, Kathy M. Kristoff, "Getting Married: Financially Speaking, A Test of Your Fiscal Compatibility," *Los Angeles Times* (February 2, 1999). © Tribune Media Service, Inc.

Pages 328, 330, "Nobody Does it Better" lyric: music by Marvin Hamlisch; lyrics by Carole Bayer Sager © 1977 DANJAQ S.A. All Rights Controlled and Administered by EMI U CATALOG INC./EMI UNART CATALOG INC. and WARNER BROS. PUBLICATIONS U.S. INC.

Photograph credits: Page 55, Spencer Tunick. All wedding photography courtesy of Debra Gerson Photography. All other photographs courtesy of the author.

A hardcover edition of ths book was published in 2004 by ReganBooks, an imprint of HarperCollins Publishers.

HarperCollins books may be purchased for educational, business,
or sales promotional use.
For information please write:
Special Markets Department, HarperCollins Publishers Inc.,
10 East 53rd Street, New York, NY 10022.

FIRST PAPERBACK EDITION PUBLISHED 2005.

Designed by Michelle Ishay and Richard Ljoenes

The Library of Congress has cataloged the hardcover edition as follows:

Lehr, Jennifer, 1969–
    Ill-equipped for a life of sex : a memoir / Jennifer Lehr.
        p. cm.
    Includes bibliographical references.
    ISBN 0-06-074157-0
        1. Lehr, Jennifer, 1969– 2. Women—Sexual behavior—Case studies. 3. Man-woman
relationships—Case studies. 4. Teenage girls—Sexual behavior—Case studies. I. Title.

HQ29.L43 2004
306.7—dc22   2004046739

ISBN 0-06-079214-0 (pbk.)

05   06   07   08   09   WBC/RRD   10   9   8   7   6   5   4   3   2   1

entirely impossible without John Lehr

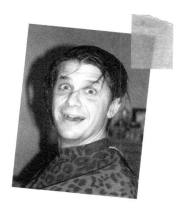

Author's Note

"At the end of a long life, one imagines the stock of secrets diminishing, for what had previously seemed an aberrant and shameful deed appears to fit more harmoniously into an understanding of what it means to be human. In this sense, the tendency of others to spill secrets may stem less from cruelty than from an ability, as an outsider, to recognize that what is deemed private in fact belongs to the province—far wider than the narrow strip the secret-holder imagines—of the normal."

—Alain de Botton, *How Proust Can Change Your Life*

My experience reminds/warns me that not one person I mention in this book will view any incident or story that I write about in remotely the same way I do. And, of course, they wouldn't/shouldn't, as there is no such thing as an objective point of view. Therefore, in the interest of trying to spare any hurt or angry feelings, I have changed most names. Unfortunately, however, when one writes a memoir, inadvertently upsetting people is virtually impossible to avoid.

contents

contents

ill-equipped for a life of sex

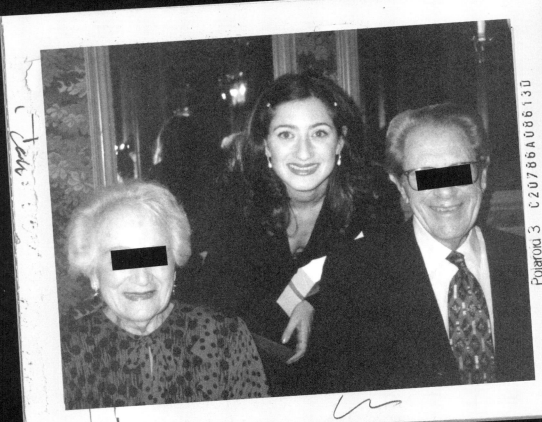

Polaroid 3 C2Û786AÛÛ613Ü

one

a granddaughter and a girlfriend

When I was the only grandchild who lived in the city (and out of the Valley), I had the distinguished privilege of serving as my grandparents' chauffeur to family events. Almost a decade later, I still haven't lost my job. And while it's not an easy position to have, it's one at which I excel. To begin with, I have to arrive exactly on time. If I'm late, I'm certainly not the granddaughter they thought I was. So, as part of my never-ending effort to make the perfect I'm-a-perfect-grandchild impression, I am always early.

Once in the car, Grandpa forbids talking because it will distract me. Should I dare try to make some polite conversation, he'll inevitably bark, "Now we're on the road, no more messing around." And, of course, the radio is totally out of the question. I won't be able to concentrate and will foolishly endanger his life more than I already am. Which I can understand. I feel sorry for him. His slowed reflexes have forced him—someone obsessed with control (well, control and money)—to put his life in my hands.

Without fail, after a bout of silence, as if Grandmother doesn't know exactly what will happen, she says something. Nothing of importance. Just something. Which means, of course, that Grandpa yells, "Honey, be quiet

Always doing my best to be the perfect grandchild.

now so she can drive." And don't think Grandpa is trying to sweeten his command with a term of endearment, because he isn't. Grandmother's *name* is Honey.

So one day, about six years ago, the three of us were driving up Pacific Coast Highway, but this time, we were talking. Maybe Grandpa allowed it because the drive was so long that we needed something to make the time pass. Or maybe he just relaxed for a minute. Whatever it was that mellowed Grandpa enough to let Grandmother open her mouth without making sure she damn well knew that her vocal cords could be the cause of his demise, she was actually able to get out both a compliment and a question.

"Jennifer, you look absolutely gorgeous today." Pause. "You are so beautiful." *Here it comes*, I thought. "Why don't you ever have a date?"

Perhaps Grandpa was so curious about the answer himself that he was willing to risk his life for the few seconds more it would take me to respond. Which I did.

"Because I don't want to upset anyone," I said stupidly. I should've just lied. But I was so excited about my new boyfriend. I was getting closer to not wanting to keep him from my family anymore.

"Because he's not Jewish?" Grandmother asked.

"Mmm-hmm."

"Well, then, you had better wait until I die to get married."

Just what I had suspected.

And then there was the day at the movies a couple of weeks later. Grandmother and I were walking down the halls of the theater when I saw a poster of a film my friend Jason had a small part in. Since she had met him recently, I said, "You remember Jason, don't you? He's in that movie." No response.

We went in and found a seat. As usual, we arrived super early, so we were just silently sitting there as slides with trivia questions about movie stars flashed on the screen, when Grandmother half turned to me and said,

"You wouldn't be stupid enough to date an actor, would you? They have no job security!"

Realizing she didn't know Jason was gay but not wanting to explain that no-no-no it was *another* non-Jewish actor I was dating—one with long hair, no less—I simply said, "Grandmother, you don't date someone because of what they do. What about love?"

Laughing angrily, she said, "Don't tell me you are so naive as to think that!"

I didn't think I was naive, but I did think I was in love. Really and finally. And despite his long hair. His name was John, and it was the height of our adorefest—what is often referred to as the "honeymoon period," a period I had waited my whole life to live. Finally, at twenty-eight years old, I was living it but afraid to tell my family that I was.

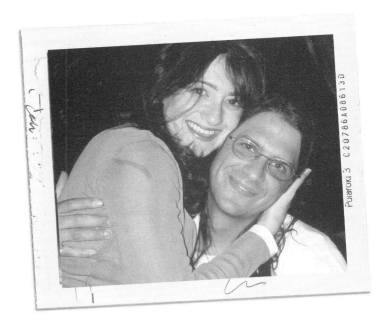

Really and finally in love—despite his long hair.

So into John was I, my ears had become especially attuned to the sound of his rusted-out, mint green, '79 Ford Grenada. Even from my fourth floor apartment, I could easily identify its rumble. As soon as I'd hear it, I'd leap up like a crazed Beatles' fan at the airport waiting for the Fab Four to deplane, inwardly shrieking, *He's here, he's finally here*! I'd rush over to my tiny iron balcony and yell down an excited "Hello, Angelhead!" and then hate the wait I'd have to endure while he put his Club on a car no one would ever steal, collected his stuff, opened the door to the building, pushed the slow old elevator's button, waited for the slow old elevator to arrive, rode up, and then finally (a whole agonizing three minutes later) landed in my arms, just where I lived for him to be.

And then six months passed and everything was a way I never could have imagined it would be. My grandparents—not one of them, *both* of them—lu-uh-uhved John. Grandmother lived for sitting in the backseat of their car with John, cuddling him every second of the drive, more than likely lamenting the life she didn't get to live with a man like John. And even my incredibly-hard-to-impress grandpa was impressed by "his boy."

And me, well, I'd had it with John by then. I was miserable. Our honeymoon period had come to an end. At first it wasn't clear. And then it was very clear. And then it was so fucking clear that John and I found ourselves driving to Beverly Hills for couples therapy.

two
muff 'n puff

Waiting in the waiting room for our fourth Tuesday-at-four-thirty couples therapy appointment with Neutral Patti, John read *Rolling Stone* while I flipped through the *Vanity Fair*. Seeing that we'd only been dating about a year and seeing that everyone thought we made such a perfect couple, our friends couldn't believe things were already so bad that we had to go.

"You're not even married!" they'd say.

"That's the point," I'd tell them, not wanting to say any more than that.

Neutral Patti opened the door and smiled hello as we walked into her office, grabbed our Evian bottles off her water shelf, and sat on the sofa in opposite spots—previously, John had always sat on my right. I made some stupid-trying-to-be-funny comment about how now things would really go differently. Neutral Patti, playing along, agreed with a polite chuckle. She got my obvious humor, but not John's. Last time he had grabbed an Arrowhead and commented how much better it tasted than Evian. Neutral P. failed to grasp his sarcasm and told him he was welcome to take whichever one he liked better.

After we sat down, I excused myself, got up, walked across the room, and picked Neutral P.'s Chapstick off the floor, explaining that I couldn't help myself, that if I left it there it would bug me the whole time—for a moment acting obsessive-compulsive in a way I'm not. It was my grasping-at-straws effort to postpone the discomfort I would feel once the session started. Neutral P. thanked me and made an equally dumb joke about how I was welcome to vacuum anytime. We were all so goddamn funny and chitchatty—that is, until our bullshit time had run out and we had no choice but to start the session in earnest.

Which meant we all sat in silence as John and I adjusted the pillows. And removed our sunglasses. And caught and averted each other's gaze. And caught Neutral Patti's and fake-smiled or lifted our eyebrows back. And crossed and uncrossed our legs. And sipped our waters. And then, after we'd done just about everything one could do on a therapist's sofa without doing the one thing we were there to do, Neutral Patti finally put us out of our who's-going-to-start-talking-first-and-about-what misery by asking us how we were.

So I told her how well we'd been getting along as John concurred with a nod. It wasn't untrue. We hadn't had one of our big fights that ended in tears and slammed doors since last week's session. However, it wasn't our progress that led to my boasting, but rather my fear of talking about what we should have been talking about. We all knew the main—though certainly not only—reason we were there. Our sex life sucked.

Somehow I mustered the nerve to inform Neutral P. that John and I showed affection differently. I explained how every time I saw John, I just wanted to kiss him and hold him and squeeze him and love him. Neutral Patti thought that was so sweet. But I knew that it was *and* it wasn't.

John explained to Neutral P. how sometimes he really liked the attention I gave him in the way I gave it to him, but sometimes (meaning more often than not) it felt like I was doing it *at* him, like he was almost incidental. In order to not waste time or money, I forced myself to admit to Neutral P. that I understood what he meant. It seemed to me, I told her, that I loved John and somehow loving him had transformed his body into this thing that I continually wanted to do "love stuff" to. Often, I'd just see him and think he was just a gorgeous pile of muff 'n puff, who has a neck that needed to be kissed, and a face that needed to be held, and a body that needed to be deeply wrapped around. At the very sight of him, I'd feel overcome with urges to touch and feel and squeeze and hold. It was like a surge inside me. *Give me that body to do with what I want!* John was saying that if I wasn't making him feel like his feelings about being squeezed were insignificant in comparison to my need to squeeze, then maybe he would want to squeeze me more.

One morning when he was in the shower, I opened the door and asked, "Angelhead, can I just give your perfect gorgeous be-hind a gentle little pinch?"

Shaking his head, he said, "I'm too wet and tired right now." And then, seeing the rejection envelop my face, he added a consolation, "How about later?"

"Okay," I said, aching with unfulfilled desire that I had to remind myself would eventually die down and go away, wishing my lover wanted to do half the stuff to me that I was dying to do to him, wondering if I'd really love it the way I imagined, or if I would tire of it like John seemed to.

What did I want? I wanted more love. What did John want? He wanted more space. And what is the one thing that will keep someone who wants more love from someone who wants more space from getting the love they want? Not giving the one who wants more space, more space. By that time in my life I certainly understood that basic relationship equation. But what I didn't understand was how John had become the one who wanted more space. Wasn't he the one who had worked so hard to win me? When had I become the chaser and he the chased? Where had the man who would open his arms to me at any given moment gone?

John, I explained to N.P., was more gentle (than I was to him and wanted him to be to me), wasn't as affectionate, and didn't have the desire to touch my body the way I did his.

"Do you think your different ways of showing affection carry over into your sex life?" N.P. cleverly asked, trying to move our discussion to the more uncomfortable place it needed to be.

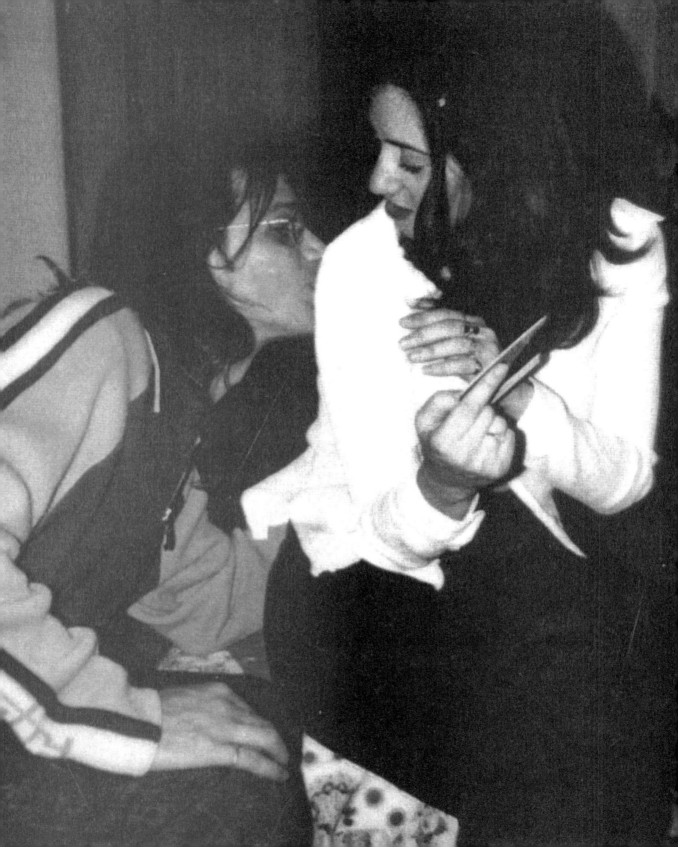

We both nodded as I muttered, "Not totally, but kind of."

And so we began. Well, we kind of began. We started to talk around stuff—not really knowing what to say, or how to get started. And I think it was hard for Neutral Patti to understand what we were saying when we did say something, so she asked us a deceptively simple question: "Which adjective would you use to best describe sex?"

What? Which adjective? I looked at her, totally confused. *A single word to describe sex?*

"What do you mean?" I asked.

So she tossed off a few examples. "You know, like 'fun' or . . ." Actually I didn't hear her second example because I instantly knew what my word was and "fun" wasn't it.

"Complicated," I said.

"Complicated," she repeated.

Then she turned to John, who started to give it some thought. As we sat there waiting for him to come up with something, I wondered how the hell N.P. could've tossed off "fun" as her example. She knew we were there precisely because it wasn't so much fun/no fun at all.

"I can't think of a word," John finally said, interrupting my internal rant about wanting a therapist who wasn't going to add insult to injury—even if it was by accident.

I was more than disappointed. I wanted to know his word. Why wasn't he trying harder? We had progress to make.

"Well, John, have you had any problems with sex in the past?" N.P. asked, trying another way in.

"Yeah, but I've always chalked it up to my drinking. But I guess since I've been sober over two years now, maybe the problems weren't only alcohol-related."

Then it was my turn to answer. "Yeah, of course I've had problems with sex," I said. *Who hasn't?* I thought. Did she really want us to recount a lifetime's worth of problems with sex? We only had two minutes left!

See? It's true. I did used to be the chased and John the chaser. Where had the man who would open his arms to me at any given moment gone?

To that end, Neutral Patti recommended double sessions every other week, explaining it would give us more time to explore things in depth. On our way out the door, N.P. informed us that she thought we had "intimacy issues." *Oh God*, I thought, *I'm in therapy for intimacy issues*. And then I thought, I *don't even know what that means!* So I asked.

"What does that mean?"

"Well, it seems to me that you both have a fear of being intimate," N.P. answered, followed by a quick, "We'll talk about it more next time."

Next time! *That's total bullshit*, I thought. *She's had four entire sessions to diagnose us and explain the diagnosis. How totally unfair to just throw that shit out at the last second like that and then close the door on us with a smile.*

Waiting for the elevator, I calmed down enough to try to think about what Neutral P. meant. I started to feel guilty that I'd been feeling so "fuck-John-for-not-fucking-me." My frustration at him started to thaw into compassion. *Who the hell do you think you are?* I scolded myself. *Miss I've-always-loved-to-fuck? When you know damn well you've spent the majority of your life plagued by a sex life you wouldn't wish on anybody?*

Whatever N.P. meant exactly, I knew she had hit something because I had felt a small wave of recognition when she said those words together: "fear" and "intimacy." After all, as a desperate-to-fit-in teenager, I had wanted nothing more than to have sex already—even though I was afraid of having it. And as a young adult, I was anxious to like the sex I was having—afraid it wouldn't happen. And then there I was, a full-fledged adult, in love with someone who now apparently had little interest in having sex with me—afraid our sex life would never improve.

What would it be like when/if John and I had sex again? How long could we go without sex and still be boyfriend/girlfriend? How was Neutral Patti going to help us?

The truth was that we hadn't had sex in two months, give or take. Well, give, definitely, give.

three

ill-equipped for sex

Before I was a desperate-to-fit-in teenager who wanted nothing more than to have sex already, I was a twelve-year-old girl with a terrible Dorothy Hamill haircut who was afraid of kissing. I was afraid of not knowing how to kiss and afraid I would never ever be kissed. My fear was rampant.

It all started with an innocent, preteen crush on a sandy-blond-haired, nasal-sounding cutie named Bobbie, who almost kissed me in seventh grade. A friend of both of ours—Rachelle—was making a short film for her film class and needed two people to run into the courtyard from opposite ends and kiss. (I went to an artsy school that was populated with kids whose parents worked in the entertainment industry, so the study of film in seventh grade wasn't unusual.) Rachelle asked me if I'd do it, explaining that I would be kissing Bobbie. Oh my God. I was so nervous. I had never kissed before. And it was Bobbie who I'd be kissing—the Bobbie I was starting to "like like."

I was so nervous that I started to make fun of the running part. Thinking I was cute and clever, I asked Rachelle if she wanted me to run like this—and then I did my best impression of the slo-mo *Chariots of Fire* run as I hummed the melodramatic theme song. I was stalling. I was terrified. Not only would it be my first kiss ever, but it would be on film! Rachelle laughed and said that she just wanted regular running.

The kiss never happened. The camera malfunctioned and the bell rang before she had a chance to fix it. For years, I was so upset about my missed opportunity. I blamed myself for screwing up the chance Rachelle had given me because I had to waste valuable time with my *Chariots of Fire* run. Perhaps if we had kissed, I'd often lament (to no one other than myself), Bobbie would've wanted to date me and my seemingly endless days and months and years of longing for him would never have had to be.

My Bobbie crush was really bad by the tenth grade, but at least I could finally admit to someone other than myself that I like-liked him. One night, when I was so tortured by my desire to be someone special to Bobbie—particularly because most of my friends all of a sudden seemed to have boyfriends—I wrote my more beautiful, mature, and experienced friend Nicole a please-help-me letter on a bunch of index cards. The next night at her house, I waited until the last second—when I heard my mom's honk—before I handed them off to her and jumped into my getaway car.

At school the next day, she handed me a folded piece of yellow legal paper that I couldn't have read fast enough or more often. It became my bible.

DUDE JEN—
Point A: You are not a geek.
Point B: Your letter is not geeky. Honesty and expression are not geeky things.
Point C: I can barely read your writing.
Point D: You are jealous? of others' fun? You may + can have it at any time. How? (SEE Point E.)
Point E: I know this may sound a bit too spiritual for you but I truly believe that once you find some security in yourself you are capable of doing and accomplishing a lot. The clothes you wear, the car you drive, the things you

say these are not aesthetically or materialistically attractive unless you find them wholly pleasing (poor sentence!). If you are pleased w/yourself (even your physical self), you are a "cool" person indeed!

Well from what I could read I found that you were feeling . . . well, sort of "boy-friendish." In other words, you find it time to get the ol' love life a chugging along. This you relay to an awesome, cute dude who wore a pink shirt and rolled pants (revealing his skinny ankles) today. I understand. I really do. Do you believe me?

Oh, and by the way, I am privileged to hear your very secret things that no one else knows about! I feel trusted etc . . . Jen, people do not know that you even care about boys and such. Therefore, people don't see you in that frame. I suppose you are not very secure in that area. And as I pointed out in "Point ë (hee hee), you need to just say "fuck it" and be the sexy-momma I know you are! for god's sakes, why don't you just go right out + say the things you think? For instance, "yeah you want to fuck this agile body?" If you said that, a few things would occur: first of all the person would be

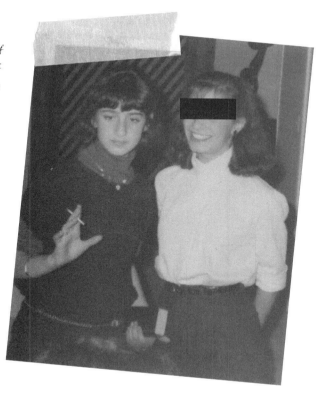

With my more beautiful, more sophisticated, and more experienced friend Neeco.

shocked, he'd then see you in a different frame. He'd see you as someone who wants "things" to happen.

Now, don't get mad—Mitch & I were talking about you one night and I mentioned that you were interested in having a boy friend, he said, "what?! really!?!" He couldn't believe it. He thought you were 100% anti-boys, sex . . . a lot of people see you like that. Many boys (Derek, Jonny, Mitch—I've talked to 'em) find you attractive yet they don't relate to you as a person having desires (gay word!). I feel that that may be the problem.

Listen up dude, this is a hell of a lot better than a 17 magazine answer! Anyway, you said "it's up to you neec," then you said you were kidding. Hey, I'll do anything I can. Dude, guys are fun—you know that. I can't believe I'd ever say this to you (perfect example of how people see you) but sex is fun. Ha! That is funny to write. Bayba, I wish you had some Dude a whole lot. You're distressed—so am I.

Damn it Jen, relax & be fun, flirty—whatever!

I love you.
—NEECO

I was at once grateful for the letter and surprised by it. I was grateful because Nicole was the first person to ever talk to me about guys and sex as if I was a grown-up with grown-up desires. But, on the other hand, I couldn't believe everyone thought I was uninterested in boys—when they all seemed to already be having sex. Why would they assume I was any different from them? *This is really getting bad*, I'd thought. *Here Nicole thinks sex is "fun" and I still haven't kissed a boy*. But she didn't know that. As far as Nicole and any of my girlfriends knew, I had kissed—at least once.

My official story was that I'd done it at summer camp, my twelve-turning-thirteen summer. Since I was lying, I could have made up anyone, but instead I chose to tell them about a guy who I really did have a thing for, who was someone I wouldn't have been proud to have kissed because he was fat. Perhaps I felt compelled to confess his size to counterbalance the lying.

Eager for their daughter to experience life beyond in suburban Los Angeles, my parents had sent me halfway across the country to Harand Camp in Elkhart Lake, Wisconsin. Billed as a theater camp, it was, in fact, a musical-theater camp where time stopped somewhere around *West Side Story*. Every building, from the cabins to the mess hall, was named after an old Broadway hit. Orientation was in the big theater, appropriately named *Our Town*, where I anxiously waited for my cabin assignment. I was distracted from my nervousness by a bunch of guys across the aisle who clearly had been to camp together before. Gosh, one was so olive-skinned and cute. And, gosh, one was so fat. Surprisingly, the fat one was the center of attention and I found myself vaguely intrigued by him.

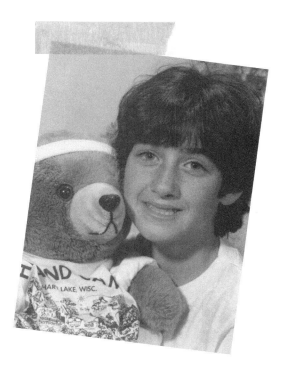

This is me the summer I *almost* kissed a boy for the first time and then just went ahead and told everyone I had.

Later I learned his name was Mickey and that he was from Las Vegas. Our first and only getting-to-know-you, grown-up-type conversation slash flirt session was on the back steps of a cabin with a small group of campers. Soon it was just the two of us. *Where did everyone go?* I wondered. *Had they sensed our attraction and left us alone?* The conversation turned to our recent Bat and Bar Mitzvahs. With some pride, I told him that my Bat Mitzvah brought me three thousand dollars. Then he nonchalantly told me he had made ten thousand. I couldn't believe it. My

Jennifer Lehr

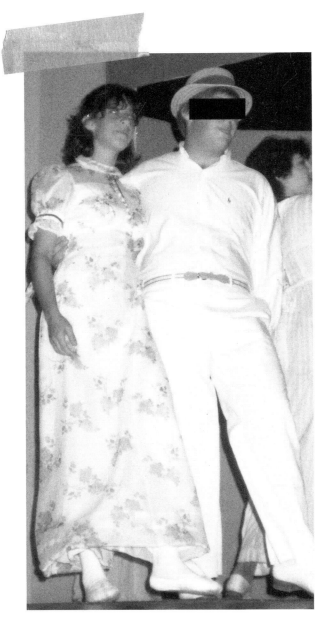

The following summer my-almost-first-kiss Mickey and I were partners in a scene in the musical *Brigadoon*. We acted as if we didn't even know each other's name. I was at once relieved and disappointed.

shock turned to shame. I was not only embarrassed that I hadn't made more myself, but that I had thought three thousand dollars was a lot of money. I was surprised to discover that despite his big nose and fat body, I was attracted to him. Maybe it was because he seemed so glamorous, what with living in Las Vegas. Or maybe because he was so funny. Or maybe it was because he made me feel like an interesting person. On the one hand, I liked that I wasn't so superficial, but on the other hand, I thought, *there's just no way*.

One night, a bunch of the *Gigi* girls planned to sneak out to meet the *South Pacific* guys at the Archery Pit. After we'd successfully made it out of our cabin and across the field to the stacks of hay without getting caught, it was as if Samantha from *Bewitched* had wiggled her nose. Instantaneously, all the kids were coupled up and making out on the ground, leaving me and Mickey standing alone, staring at each other.

I had never snuck out before and was amazed at how it was understood by everyone what we were there to do. Because there were the same

16

number of girls and boys, I wondered how everyone already knew I'd be with Mickey. I'd never even mentioned him to anyone, yet apparently everyone knew and he knew and I knew that he knew. But how? Just because we talked on the steps about our Bar Mitzvahs? As he walked toward me I thought, *Why does the first guy I'm going to kiss have to be fat? What will people think of me getting together with a fat kid even though he's a cool fat kid? Did this mean we'll have to make out every day? Will I want to? Am I not cute enough to get a cuter guy?*

With another wiggle from Samantha's nose, Mickey was sitting cross-legged and I was lying on my back with my head in his lap. I took one last look at the stars and resigned myself to my fate as Mickey leaned down to kiss me. Just as the heat of his opening mouth hit my face, I whispered, "Wait. I have to take my retainer out." Stalling, I got up, walked past the making-out couples, and put it on top of a haystack for safekeeping, as I said to myself, *Okay, this is it. No more excuses. Now, right now, is going to be your first kiss.* I lay back down. And then, just when Mickey was back with his big nose and ruddy cheeks just inches from my trying-to-remain-calm face, the flashlights came. We were in big trouble. As we followed our counselors back to our cabin, I said, "Wait, I forgot my retainer."

And that's the story I told my girlfriends—minus the not-kissing part. I'd just explain that, after I took my retainer off, we made out like everyone else. I stuck to that lie for three long, torture-filled years. Each time I told it I became more humiliated that I still hadn't kissed a guy—that I still had to tell the Mickey story. *What was tongue-kissing like?* I wondered. Anxious to be able to disguise myself as someone who'd already kissed when the moment came, I was constantly staring at people who did it publicly to learn whatever I could. I didn't want the guy who was going to be my first kiss to know he was, because I assumed if he knew, he'd think there was something wrong with me, something like I wasn't attractive or worth kissing because, if I was, then surely I would've already been kissed.

One night, while at my aunt's for Passover dinner, a thirteen-year-old me went in to check on my already-sleeping, adorable toddler cousin Mark with the blond curly locks. Seeing him there with his mouth slightly open—all

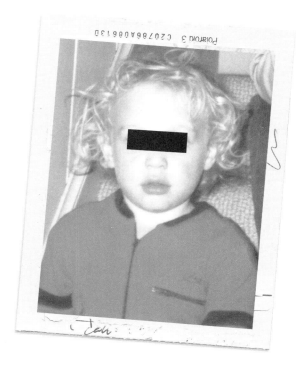

This is my innocent cousin Mark who I wanted to practice French-kissing on.

slimy like little baby mouths are—I thought, *This is my chance. I've got to try it.* So eager was I to know what someone's tongue would feel like against mine, I leaned down to give him a kiss. But I stopped. I couldn't do it. Fortunately, I had the presence of mind to think, *You can't French-kiss a sleeping three-year-old! That's sexual molestation. You'll ruin his whole life.*

Meanwhile, I continued my relentless pursuit of Bobbie in what I had hoped was a very unassuming way. At school it wasn't so easy because he had his group of guy friends, but after school I would call . . . a lot. Fortunately for my obsession, he had his own line—rare in those days. I alternated my excuses for calling. There was the homework excuse and the wrong-number excuse. Sometimes I would combine them:

"Hello, wait, who's this?"

"Bobbie."

"Oh God, Bobbie, sorry, I was trying to call Nicole, your numbers are so similar."

"That's okay."

"Hey, have you done the math homework yet?" I'd ask in an attempt to get a conversation going. Sometimes I was successful.

I also did stuff like making sure I picked a country in Africa that was close to the country Bobbie had already picked for our Socials Studies report. That way he might want to borrow my books on the region. Meanwhile, he always had girlfriends. At fifteen, he was seeing a girl with dyed blond hair from another school, whom he was always driving around on his Vespa. It killed me. What did they do together? And why didn't he want to do it with me? *Why*, I wondered, *would I feel attracted to someone if he wasn't going to feel it back? Didn't my feeling feelings for someone mean we were supposed to be together?*

My first real kiss finally happened the summer my friend Derek and I got our driver's licenses. Just before our birthdays rolled around, we had several just-friends nights that were charged—preparation nights that said a kiss could very well be coming soon.

Like Mickey, Derek was overweight. And it didn't escape me that the first guy I'd almost kissed and the first guy I might kiss were not the thin cuties I longed for. While I wondered why the funniest, most fun, smartest, and most interested-in-me guys had to have extra fat on their bodies, what I really wondered was, *Would I be able to handle caressing Derek's chubbiness should things get that far?*

One preparation night, Derek and I got superstoned out my bathroom window and ran around my bedroom in our underpants playing "bull and conquistador." Apparently, my parents thought nothing of our sleepovers. It was as if they thought I was still ten and Derek was one of my girlfriends. Little did they know, Derek had first had sex at thirteen—with a redheaded bombshell on the beach! I was intimidated by his experience.

Should my parents have given me some kind of sex talk before they let him sleep over? Something about how I might feel like I want to do stuff and it's okay to feel it and to not do it, or okay to feel it and do some stuff but to feel confident about saying when I thought enough was enough? Would it have helped me to have the confidence to tell guys what I was really feeling? Would it have helped me tell my parents what I was really feeling? Well, fortunately, I didn't need the talk they didn't give me (that I was relieved not to have had to squirm through) because Derek and I were so worn-out from all of our charging and grazing that we passed out with the lights on—he in his tighty whities and me in some skimpy look.

Another preparation night, we pretended to be engrossed in the TV as our hands screwed for what seemed like hours—our fingers twisting, pushing, pulling, rubbing, and squeezing. Pot gave us the courage.

Finally, Derek's patience and my fear both gave way after yet another preparation night of driving around, smoking pot, and singing to Fleetwood Mac and Led Zeppelin. Sitting in his car in front of my house, we exhausted every topic I could think of. With no stalls left in my arsenal, I said good night, got out of his car, came around to his side to give him a hug, and casually leaned against the car as I eked out one more thing to say. I knew that within seconds we'd be kissing. But I was afraid. Afraid of seeming so glaringly inexperienced and afraid of formally acknowledging—via our kiss—that there was more than friendship between us.

It wasn't like I thought it would be. Derek didn't open his mouth and flutter his tongue with mine. It was slower and mushier. He did smaller, gentler stuff that I wasn't prepared for. But I was kissing! As I tried to do what he was doing, I worried that my parents might come to the window to check if I was home and see me doing adultlike stuff. I couldn't imagine admitting to them that I had a crush or that I was dating. We didn't talk about that stuff—ever.

As soon as there was room for a breath, I said good night and quickly ran into the house, thrilled with my success and beyond relieved. I'd finally done it. My mini-celebration, however, abruptly came to a halt when I realized that the kiss meant that we'd probably do it again. I somehow instantly knew that I didn't want to "go out" with Derek. And it wasn't because I didn't adore him. It was because I was afraid of having to "go further" with him. I just wanted to have kissed someone so that I didn't feel like I hadn't, and everyone else had, and that no one wanted to kiss me. At the same time, however, I was curious about learning to do the stuff my girlfriends were doing. I didn't want to be left behind. I didn't want to be thought of as a prude.

I was relieved when Derek called to tell me that his friend Larry—who'd graduated two years earlier—would be joining us for our next night out. The pressure was off. After hours spent parked at the beach getting high, looking at the moon, talking about life, and fancying ourselves particularly deep thinkers, we dropped Larry at his house. Seeing that we had another twenty minutes before we got to mine, I comfortably slouched my stoned self down in the seat, put my feet on the dash, and closed my eyes as we curved our way east on Sunset Boulevard. I don't know how Derek knew that it was okay to do this, but soon he reached over and started rubbing an area of me that I had never referred to out loud.

As a little girl, it was an area that I can only remember my mother referring to as "my crotch," a surprisingly vague term considering that as the curriculum director of the elementary school she owned with my dad, she had instituted a sex-education program that was very cutting-edge for the seventies. While my mother is certainly to be commended for making sure her daughter—and hundreds of other children—were educated about things she undoubtedly was not educated about in the 1940s, the classes didn't make it any easier for my mother and me to discuss things like boys, kissing, or calling my vagina a vagina.

So Derek was rubbing a part of me that not only had never been rubbed, but that I didn't feel comfortable identifying. And it felt amazing. He somehow managed to take unlit hairpin curve after hairpin curve along Sunset Boulevard while continuing to rub me and rub me as the throbbing intensified exponentially. When he pulled up at my house, I acted too tired to do any making out. I just scurried off, afraid, wondering what I was afraid of. I couldn't make sense of how it was that when I was a little girl, I played lots of sex games with my friends and wasn't afraid—beyond being afraid of being caught by our retired-nun housekeeper who would be sure to spank me if she caught me once again playing naked with a friend in the closet. But now that I was at an age when I was supposed to do sex stuff (evidenced by all the stuff my friends were doing), why was I so nervous and so not up for it? *Where*, I wondered, *has my childhood sexual confidence gone?*

At three years old, I was on fire—a daring little sexpot whose big idea it was to have sex with my friend Adam one afternoon while our mothers ate lunch. According to plan, we went into my room, took off our clothes, and sat on the floor. After a few minutes of staring down at our naked private parts, confused about how we were going to do what we'd set out to, we

Jennifer Lehr

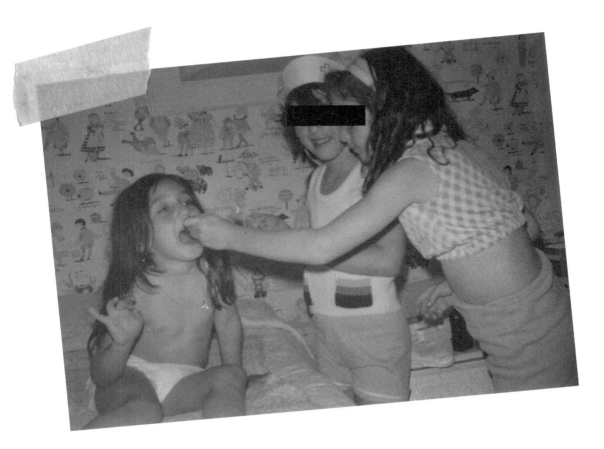

Playing good
old-fashioned
doctor.

had no choice but to abort our plans. We simply couldn't figure it out. But it was just the beginning of a burgeoning sexual relationship between us.

We loved playing Insect Inspector in the tree house. Lying on my belly, I'd busy myself inspecting the floor for insects while Adam (for some unexplained reason) would pull my pants down, little by little, as I pretended not to notice. It was incredibly arousing. After my pants were all the way down, we'd act like it never happened and then we'd switch. I preferred being the insect inspector, which meant I liked being the one inspected. Adam was just one of my many young sex-game partners and Insect Inspector was just one game among other favorites, like Nude Model, Boyfriend/Girlfriend, and, of course, good old-fashioned Doctor.

So there I was, at sixteen, jealous of my fearless sexuality as a little kid. Despite my anxiety, Derek and I had a few more encounters that made me feel like a grown-up with a private life. However, I soon discovered, kissing was one thing—doing other stuff was another. One day, when Derek pulled over to make out, he reclined my seat back, lifted my shirt up, and started sucking on my breasts. I felt suffocated but tried my best to participate. I wanted to want to pull over and kiss, I just didn't want to. So after he dropped me off, I decided I had to avoid Derek. It was too much, too fast with someone too fat.

Confused by my silence, he wrote me a note—my first from a boy:

> A lot has happened in the last few weeks. We don't talk about it. I wonder why. I can't tell how you feel, and that throws me. I don't know what this has all been to you . . .

I didn't either! I couldn't handle the increasing amount of sexual activity, which I never could have brought myself to tell him. I desperately wanted to be able to go back to being nonkissing friends who loved hanging out, getting stoned, and singing at the top of our lungs together. I didn't respond to his note and just hoped the problem would somehow go away before school started.

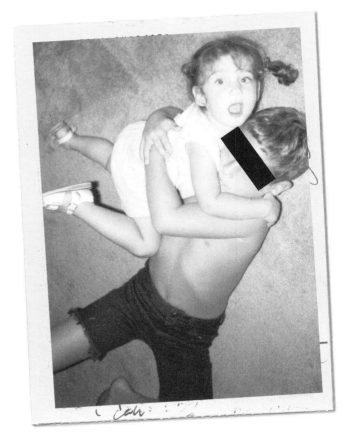

Back in the heyday of my sexual confidence, playing with one of my many young sex-games partners.

Meanwhile, Derek's pothead friend Larry called to see if I wanted to go to a movie. Which I did. Starting a new relationship was much easier than attending to one that needed sorting out. Our unofficial date ended on my twin bed, making out with his hard penis pushing against my thigh. Encouraging myself to just go ahead and try it, I unbuckled his belt, scooted my hand down his tight Levi's, grabbed ahold, and started to rub.

"Too hard! Be more gentle," Larry loudly whispered to a mortified me. It couldn't have been more clear that I'd never done before what I was attempting to do then. As I did my best to follow his instructions, Larry said, "You haven't had sex before, have you?"

"No," I admitted.

"Do you want to?" he asked, as if it was obvious that I was long past due—which I thought I was. It seemed that every one of my best girlfriends had not only had sex, but liked it. Nicole thought it was "fun." Lauren couldn't wait for her after-school "dates" with Johnny, when they'd try out the next position from their book on sex positions. Wendy bragged about doing it on the roof of a rock club, and in another hole no less! Carrie went back to Gregg's house during their free periods to do it. And even little Hillary did it with Jason—as far as I could guess without actually having the nerve to ask. Hell yes, I wanted to do it.

"Yeah, I guess so," I said as he kissed me.

Unlike Derek, Larry was thin and he lived out of town, which means he was—both my conscious and subconscious agreed—a viable candidate as a devirginizer because no matter what happened, I wouldn't have to deal with it.

"We can go down to my parents' place in Newport Beach," he offered.

"Okay," I said.

"How about Tuesday?" he asked.

Tuesday afternoon, I put on my favorite dress, the one with a tight white tank top that extended down past my hip bones before it flared out. I wore white ballet slippers and a brown leather bomber jacket, and loved my look.

I picked Larry up in my dad's black Mustang convertible with red leather interior and off we went to sit in typical stop-and-go traffic, breathing in the heavy smog every inch of the way. What should have taken forty-five minutes took over two hours, but seemed like an eternity to an anxious-but-desperately-trying-to-play-it-cool me.

As soon as we arrived, Larry wanted to get stoned. I didn't, but took the pipe when he handed it to me. Then we climbed up the ladder to the loft. Eager to get it over with, I bravely started to touch Larry's neck and shoulder, and then leaned in for a kiss that wasn't returned.

"Not so fast," Larry said, chastising me. Clearly, he had a particular way he had envisioned deflowering me, and my taking some initiative wasn't part of it.

Rejected and stoned, I soon found myself lying limply on my back, my legs slightly spread, with his pasty white body weighing down on me as he struggled to put his penis into the right place. I was surprised when it was over so quickly because I didn't feel the pain I'd heard about. Actually, it didn't feel like much. Larry was too consumed with how he wanted me to experience having sex for the first time to notice how I was actually experiencing it. Twenty minutes later, we were on the beach smoking Marlboro reds, finally doing something I loved.

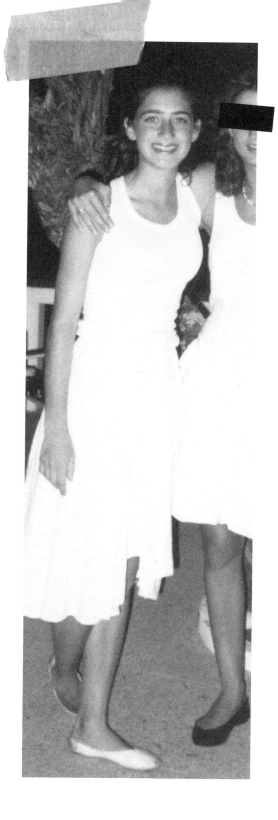

Appropriately, I wore white to my devirginization.

"How do you feel?" he asked.

"I don't know." I shrugged, annoyed by the question, grateful for my cigarette. But I knew. I was relieved. Relieved I'd done it and relieved Larry lived in New York.

The best news, however, was that my plan had worked. All along I had suspected that Bobbie would finally find me attractive once I was more experienced. And I was right.

It was a still-early-in-my-senior-year night when, once again, and like so many times before, I'd managed to bullshit my way over to Bobbie's house for some homework reason. After our official business was done, he walked me to my car in the dark and said, "You've had sex before, haven't you?"

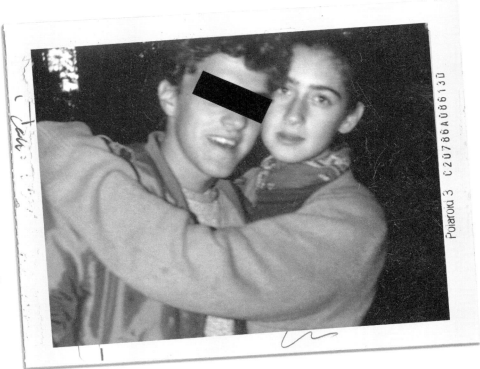

For ten minutes, I'd finally got my Bobbie. Though our first make-out was incredible, trying to suck him off in the backseat of a car sucked.

"Oh yeah," I said, as nonchalantly as I could, as I proudly patted myself on my back.

Hearing my news, Bobbie proceeded to kiss me. And I loved it. It was truly my first I-like-how-this-feels make-out session. He lifted my favorite muted gold lace skirt, and squeezed my barely-covered-by-my-even-lacier-green-string-bikini ass, and kissed me hard. We opened our mouths wide and our tongues dove deep. I drove home ecstatic, triumphant—certain that now we'd finally, some six years into my infatuation, go out.

The next week, I found myself in the backseat of the Volvo station wagon that Bobbie's housekeeper drove, trying not to gag as I attempted to suck his penis at his clumsy request. Not remotely interested in actually looking at it, I quickly put it in my mouth and closed my eyes and tried to do what Jennifer Jason Leigh did to that carrot at the mall in *Fast Times at Ridgemont High*. I was so relieved they'd put that educational scene in the movie. Otherwise, how would I have known what to do? Blow jobs weren't the kind of thing covered in our school's pathetic attempt at sex education.

In all of my years at my junior high/high school, I only recall one science class devoted to the discussion of sex. And the class wasn't so much about sex as it was about birth control. It was almost as if it was accepted that we were all screwing, so they (the educators) just wanted to make sure we knew our options. And, of course, it speaks volumes that the school thought sex should be addressed in science class in the first place. Talking about sex through the lens of reproduction, and throwing in safety precautions for good measure, ensured that feelings on the subject would never be addressed. And our school was so much more progressive than most schools. They even offered psychology in twelfth grade—albeit as an elective. But, of course, that class was still very dryly academic and not remotely do-you-ever-wonder-why-you-might-be-attracted-to-whom-you-are-attracted-to? I think I would've perked up to some relevant questions as opposed to trying to stay awake during an explanation of the id.

Jennifer Lehr

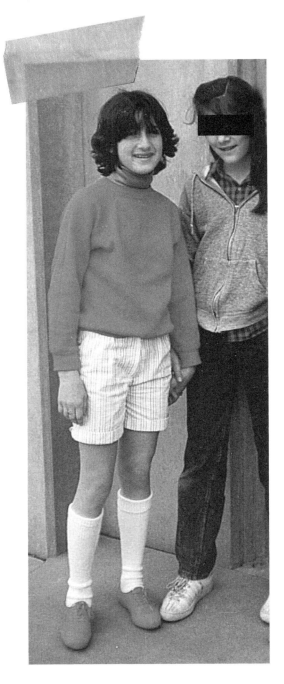

Best friends since seventh grade, it was over for Lauren and me. Turns out Bobbie wanted to sleep with her instead of me, even though she was his best friend's girlfriend.

What the school had was a crisis on its hands, a crisis that they were not only totally ill-equipped to manage, but apparently one to which they were totally oblivious. Here they had a school full of kids, half of whom had divorced parents/terrible role models for relationships, doing an inordinate amount of cocaine, ecstasy, speed, and pot—and having sex under not-the-best-of-conditions.

As it turned out, Bobbie and I wouldn't be dating. He ended up secretly, and then not so secretly, sleeping with my best friend, Lauren, who was also his best friend Johnny's girlfriend. While everyone in our class was aghast at how Lauren could do this to Johnny (leaving Bobbie virtually blame-free), I wondered how she could do this to me. She knew I was in love with Bobbie. I was devastated. Best friends since seventh grade, it was over for us.

As I tried to come to terms with the fact that I was now too old to ever experience the ecstasy of "puppy love," like Molly Ringwald did in *Sixteen Candles* or Brooke Shields did in *The Blue Lagoon*, I reassured myself that in college I would finally fall in love and have a real, honest-to-goodness boyfriend. Finally, all of my wanting to do it/not wanting to do it, rejecting/being rejected would be over. I was going to be loved and normal, because I was normal and lovable.

In retrospect, it's surprising that I—a smart and perceptive kid—was so totally convinced that I was the only one not telling the truth about my private life. Did my girlfriends really love sex as much as they claimed to, or, more than likely, did we not have the confidence, the trust, and the vocabulary to honestly talk about sex with each other? Even now, my thirty-year-old girlfriends and I don't do such a hot job of being educated, liberated, sophisticated women, comfortable with our sexuality, who can freely talk about sex.

four

assessing

Because my sex life with John was not what I was hoping it would be, I was always trying to figure out what my friends' sex lives were like, to see where John and I fit in.

There was my friend Daniella and her boyfriend, Sam—who she'd never thought was bright enough, but who did place her sufficiently high on a pedestal. Their problems were nothing I could relate to. Daniella complained that Sam wanted to screw up to three times a day(!) and she just didn't feel like doing it all the time. Listening closely, I didn't hear her say she didn't want to do it at all. It sounded to me like she did like doing it, but not that often. Our conversation kind of stopped there. Sam wanted to have as much sex in a single day as John wanted to have in six months.

For a straight-male point of view, there was my single-for-the-first-time-in-a-long-while friend Paul, who had recently flown up to San Francisco to shoot a "porno" with a woman he used to date. His report was that it was as erotic and hot as he'd hoped—definitely worth the price of the plane ticket. Selfishly, I hadn't wanted to hear too much about it, because I knew that the details would further depress me about my and John's lack of experimentation . . . well, our lack of sex in general—forget experimentation.

Paul returned to L.A. to go out with an old friend, who, at the end of the evening, interrupted their kiss to lament the bad timing. She had a boyfriend, to tell him the truth. *Aggh*, I thought, instantly identifying with the girl. I didn't want to go out with a male friend only to find myself dying to kiss him, forcing myself not to, going home to be with John who wouldn't want to kiss me, and then plummeting further into my misery.

Then there was my gay friend Jason. Single and sexual as all get-out, at dinner he could barely take his eyes off our handsome waiter to listen to a thing I had to say. Jason said he was so horny that he could fuck the prep cooks we could see working in the kitchen. At the time, Jason was—on occasion—having amazingly hot sex with a closeted married man at a hotel by the airport. He was also having some very interesting nights hanging out (in a hot tub or by a fire) with "for-the-record" straight guys who wanted to try some stuff while hopped up on other stuff. Stuff like having their cocks sucked while out of their minds on methamphetamines or some such inhibition-dropping drug.

(I was so busy being jealous of Daniella's horny boyfriend, Paul's porno, and Jason's exciting nights that I didn't realize that I wasn't as alone as I'd thought. I didn't notice that this fear of intimacy was everywhere. Daniella's boyfriend's sex obsession was driving her away. Paul was having great sex with someone in another city and was going on dates with some- one who had a boyfriend. Jason was fucking men who wouldn't admit to being gay, who needed drugs to make out. While certainly my friends were having a hell of a lot more sex than I was, they weren't getting closer to anyone.)

I was relieved when I found a friend with sex problems I could relate to. After more than a couple of gently probing e-mails, Meredith and I admit- ted our embarrassing predicaments to each other. Maybe the three thou- sand miles away we lived from each other helped. From what I could glean, Mer and her husband, Michael, had problems similar to ours, but in re- verse. Like John, Mer seemed to have lost her interest in sex.

She confessed a fight she and Michael had had not too long after returning from their fabulous European honeymoon. An I-can't-take-this-rejection-from-my-new-bride-another-minute Michael was desperately trying to get Mer to tell him why she no longer found him attractive—as if she actually knew. Since their problems certainly predated his proposal, Mer yelled back, "Well, then, why did you marry me?"

"Because *that's* how much I love you."

So while it was a relief that Mer and Michael were suffering, too, I certainly didn't want to ever find myself married to a John who still didn't want to fuck me. And weren't sex lives not supposed to disintegrate until after marriage?

There's nothing like turning on *Oprah* for some assurance that you're not alone. One day John had come home while I was watching, and he sat down to watch with me. Oprah's guest was Christina Ferrare, who had, apparently, shocked the world (or a lot of women at home in the afternoon with their TVs on) when she'd confessed her lack of sexual desire on a previous show. Ferrare's admission spawned an onslaught of letters from viewers thanking her for her honesty. Like her, they thought they were the only ones feeling that way. The overwhelming responses inspired her new book, entitled *Okay, So I Don't Have a Headache*. And now she was back to promote it. Needless to say, I was interested in a show about not wanting to have sex with your mate. Was John?

In her introduction, Oprah explained Christina lost interest in sex when she was in her late forties . . . so I was still interested, but John wasn't pre-menopausal and certainly wouldn't ever be. This wasn't the show for us. But we (I had the remote) stayed through the commercials. Oprah's next two guests who complained of a serious decline in their sexual desire were closer in age to us. They were women, of course. What man is going to go on *Oprah* with that admission, right?

So we stayed tuned and heard this twenty-eight-year-old talk about how she had always had great sex with her now husband before they were married, but then, soon after she became his wife, she suddenly found she

didn't want to do it anymore, and was plagued by guilt and feelings of failure. Since she was desperate not to lose her husband, her solution was to
designate certain days as Sex Days, days at the end of which she would definitely make sure she had "made love" with her husband. All Sex Day long,
she would try to mentally prepare her anxiety-ridden self for the task she
hated herself for dreading. She said that once she was actually engaging in
the sex, it was okay, or maybe even good, I don't remember. It was the
anticipation of doing what she thought she had to do to save her marriage
that was so excruciating. Broaching the subject with her partner for life—
who surely deeply loved and cared for her—never seemed to have crossed
her mind.

I sat there wondering what John thought of all this. Was that similar to
how he felt? I mustered the nerve to ask him a question, trying to use my
best let's-have-a-mellow-discussion-about-this voice so he wouldn't feel
uncomfortable or become defensive.

"Angelhead, can you relate to any of this?"

"No," he said.

So I turned off the TV. No discussion. On with our day. While Oprah was
vaguely reassuring, she wasn't helpful. John wasn't remotely ready to talk
about his feelings and I wasn't remotely able to help him.

Oprah wasn't our only source for sex on TV. We were fans of *Sex and the
City*. We'd been glued to several segments of HBO's *Real Sex*. We'd seen the
one on sex workers. The one contrasting various cultural attitudes toward
sex, that featured Japanese men who bought used girls' underwear from
vending machines. The one on swinging. The one on role-playing. The one
with explicit how-to tips that featured a room full of women who you
might've thought were at a Tupperware party but instead were at a learn-
how-to-suck-dick party—a party which, I might add, I did not need to attend. We'd flip channels late at night and every so often find ourselves
paused on porn stations. Sometimes I'd get turned on and sometimes so
would he. *If he's hard, why doesn't he want to do something about it?* I'd wonder,

turning over angry, not wanting to risk making another advance that more than likely wouldn't be returned. I'd lie there angry. And I'd wake up angry.

The constant rejection from John had drained all sympathy from my body. It was as if I had amnesia, and didn't remember that I, too, had acutely suffered from a fear of talking about my problems with sex. I'm sure my first semi-real boyfriend, Dylan, remembers my silence well. He couldn't have been more patient, loving, or caring, and yet I couldn't manage to discuss, admit, or reveal a goddamned thing. Wondering what I should say to John to jump-start our communication on the topic, I tried to think what Dylan should've said to me to help me be less afraid of telling him why I didn't want to have sex with him.

five

Unfortunately for me, Dylan was not the first guy I met at college. It would take a couple of more-than-uncomfortable messes before I'd find my way to him. They were the kind of messes that Neutral P. would surely submit as evidence of her fear of intimacy theory. And in retrospect, I'd have to agree.

Double unfortunately, socializing at Connecticut College revolved around keg parties. I hated beer and I hated kegs. Metal vats of piss-colored foam? And beer bongs? This form of "socializing" was new to me. I was more used to trying to be cool via smoking a joint or doing a line of coke, but kegs? I didn't get it. If one was going to drink alcohol, wouldn't one prefer to do it using a martini glass? New to the East Coast, I figured I had no choice but to try to adapt.

During my first week, it was at a "keg" on the "quad" that I met a sophomore named Nick. He was tallish, sandy-blondish, and fluttered his bloodshot eyes when he talked. I thought his nervous tic made him sexy—why, I don't know. Of all the guys drinking beer on the quad, this is the one I felt drawn to. He flirted with me and I flirted with him, which led me to believe: *This is the guy. He's going to be my first true boyfriend*. That's how I thought it happened. After all, I'd been in *South Pacific* at Harand

Camp singing, "Some enchanted evening . . . you may see a stranger, you may see a stranger . . . [band swells] across a crowded room, and somehow you know, you know even then . . . that somewhere you'll see [him] again and again."

And I did. I thought I knew, that I knew even then, that he was my true love whom I'd be seeing again and again. The enchanted evening with the stranger from across the crowded quad ended in his cinder-block dorm room with me recommending we use a condom—a recommendation that wasn't easy for me to muster the courage to whisper. He dutifully grabbed one and gave it to me to put on. Oh God, I'd never done that before. I handed it back, indicating he should do it, embarrassed by my inexperience. After we did it . . . or, rather, after he did it to me, he thought it best if I went back to my dorm.

And then, even then, I thought I knew I'd see him again and again. Which I did. But not because he wanted to see me. I became obsessed with the Eye Flutterer that first college semester. Trying to be nonchalant, I continually stopped by his room in a casual hey-I-just-happened-to-be-in-your-dorm way. The Eye Flutterer was my Bobbie at college. Subconsciously, pining was uncomfortably comfortable for me. Being in an actual relationship was unimaginable.

During this pining-for-the-Eye-Flutterer time, I found myself, curiously often, visiting the second floor of my dorm, hanging out with my newfound sophomore friend Pete. While Pete was boyishly cute and had a charm about him, for some inexplicable reason, I didn't consider him boyfriend material. Sometimes our long talks ended with me on top of him, rocking away. "Dry-humping" was the term I later heard derisively used to describe this behavior (by a guy who wanted me to let him wet-fuck me). But Pete and I never kissed. We didn't remove clothes. We didn't fondle or grope. We simply talked and dry-humped.

Our strange behavior took me as much by surprise as it did Pete. One day hanging out in his room talking—him on his bed, me on a chair—led to both of us lying on his bed talking, which led to lying on his bed feeling incredibly turned on and struggling to keep a conversation going as if nothing else was happening. But then suddenly, so turned on did I feel that day, I rolled myself on top of him and started to push my pelvis into his belly. And then I couldn't think straight. All I could do was keep pushing because that indescribable feeling demanded I did. A few rocks back and forth later, everything came to a grinding halt. The dark hole of sexual ecstasy had vanished and I found myself stuck in an ugly dorm room wanting nothing more than to leave. Which I did, with an awkward "See you later." And as I did, I wondered if I'd just had an orgasm. It's not like I was screaming or groaning. But maybe, yeah. I guess that's what happened.

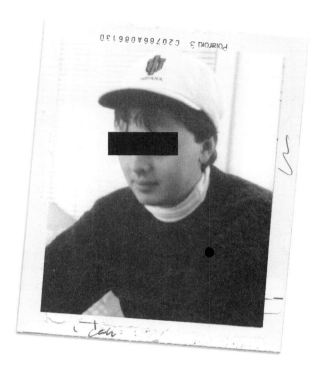

This is Pete, my dry-humping partner.

These "hump" sessions became more routine, though it wasn't something we ever formally acknowledged. Eventually, however, Pete did say, "This really is odd, you know." Mortified by the acknowledgment, and confused by what the hell my body felt so compelled to have me do, I never let it happen again.

Now, my time at school wasn't only spent dry-humping Pete and occasionally getting screwed and screwed over by the Eye Flutterer. I saw myself as a relatively normal undergrad who had an easy time adjusting to college life. I loved my modern-dance classes to live drums in the enormous glass-walled studio, with views of a grove of evergreens. I felt particularly collegiate when attending my Philosophy 101 and English-literature classes in the imposing limestone building overlooking the vast lacrosse fields and Long Island Sound. I wrote solid papers on the new Macintosh Grandmother had bought me. *Ich Deutsch sprechen* at 9 A.M. every morning. I was getting A's and B's. I loved being away from home so I could smoke freely and often. I liked the friends I was making. I loved the oatmeal cookies in the lounge. I didn't gain the freshman fifteen. School was good. It was my sex/lack-of-love life that plagued me.

Another sophomore named Patrick was the next guy to make me less than proud of how I was handling my new life as a young, attractive, sexually active woman-in-the-making. A bit of a nerd and very Bostonian in his khakis, polo shirts, and tortoiseshell glasses, Patrick was tall, awkward, gentle, and smitten. And he was a virgin. A male sophomore virgin! I sympathized with his condition. Almost unable to bear what I assumed was his humiliation and curiosity another minute, I offered to help out. How was he to know that I was so totally ill-equipped for the job?

Removing his boxers, Patrick lay down on his too-little-for-such-a-long-guy twin dorm bed. Barely able to look at what he'd just revealed, I stole a glance and was relieved to find that he was already hard, so all I had to do was lift up my skirt, move my panties to the side, and sit on his erection. Joylessly rocking back and forth If thought, *Fuck, why did I start this? He doesn't seem to be getting excited. Who would be? What should I do? Oh God, I've made things worse. His first fuck might just be a terrible, loused-up attempt. Please come. Please come.* Fortunately, he did and I was so relieved. What the fuck was I doing as a devirginizer? More than empathy was required for the undertaking.

And only then did Dylan, out of nowhere, save me from myself.

We met thanks to a project I was doing for my sculpture class. The assignment was entitled "An Investigation of Repetition of Form." We had to create a sculpture using at least seven of the same object. And I don't know how I got it, but a strange and rather grandiose idea came to me. Was it a good idea? I couldn't tell. Would I look stupid in front of everyone when it was time to share my sketch? With my heart pounding and my voice shaking, I explained that the lacrosse fields would be my canvas and Volkswagen Bugs would be my form. After hearing idea after idea—most of which involved

Coke bottles and pillows—it was clear that my idea was, by far, the most original. My professor was impressed and I was excited.

I'd always thought of myself as an artist and now I was starting to fancy myself very avant-garde. I developed a romanticized notion of myself as a young Christo who would shake up my rather conservative school by parking so many VW Bugs in the center of the campus. I approached my project with a fervor I thought matched that of the Dadaists in 1920s Berlin about whom I'd been reading. I was enamored of their rebellious spirit and sense of the absurd. I'd get those cars onto that snowy field with their engines roaring and their horns honking at the start of a school day if it was the last thing I did. On my dot-matrix printer, I printed out my appeal letter—*Dear Bug Owner . . . I would like to borrow your Bug for one hour at 9* A.M. *. . .* —which I put on the windshield of all the Bugs I could find both on campus and off. Nervously, I waited to hear from their owners.

Among those who responded was Dylan, a senior with a red Bug. Intrigued, he wanted to meet for lunch to hear more about my project. Sitting at a corner table in a dorm dining room I'd never ventured into before, I animatedly told him about all the problems I'd been having getting permission from the college to drive the cars onto the school's beloved lacrosse and soccer fields: "Security told me to talk to maintenance and maintenance told me to talk to the dean of student life, who told me to talk to maintenance." I carried on as if I were curing cancer. And he listened with great interest. Lunch was fun and Dylan asked if I wanted to meet for lunch again tomorrow.

We proceeded to have lunch together, every single day, for three months straight. Lunchtime was the highlight of my life. One day, after discussing which dorm we wanted to dine in the next afternoon, Dylan asked me if I wanted to join him for dinner that very night. Finally, a boyfriend who was going to love me for me. But because there always had to be something that kept me from being able to fully embrace the relationship, this time I recoiled/tried not to recoil from his slightly pockmarked skin.

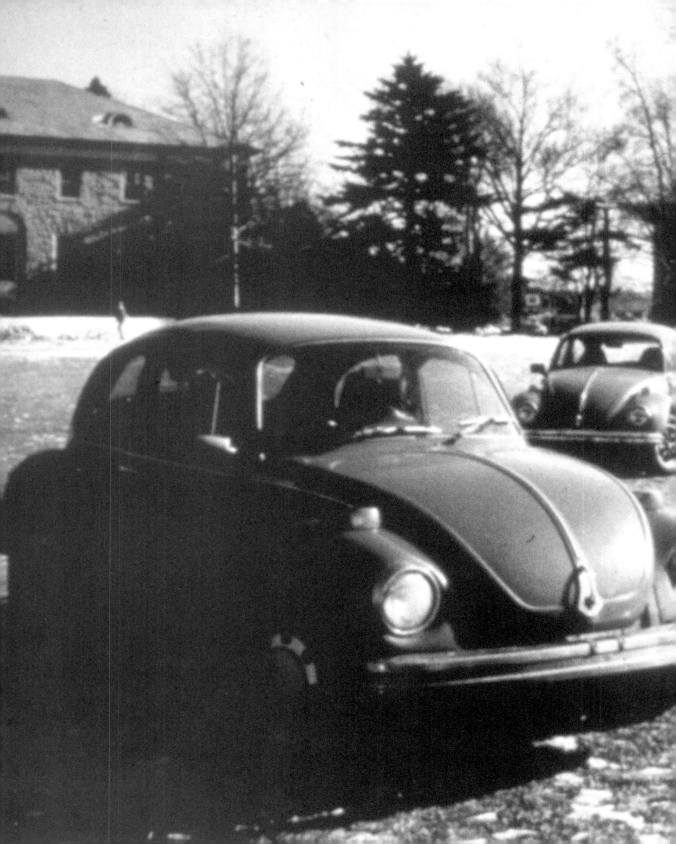

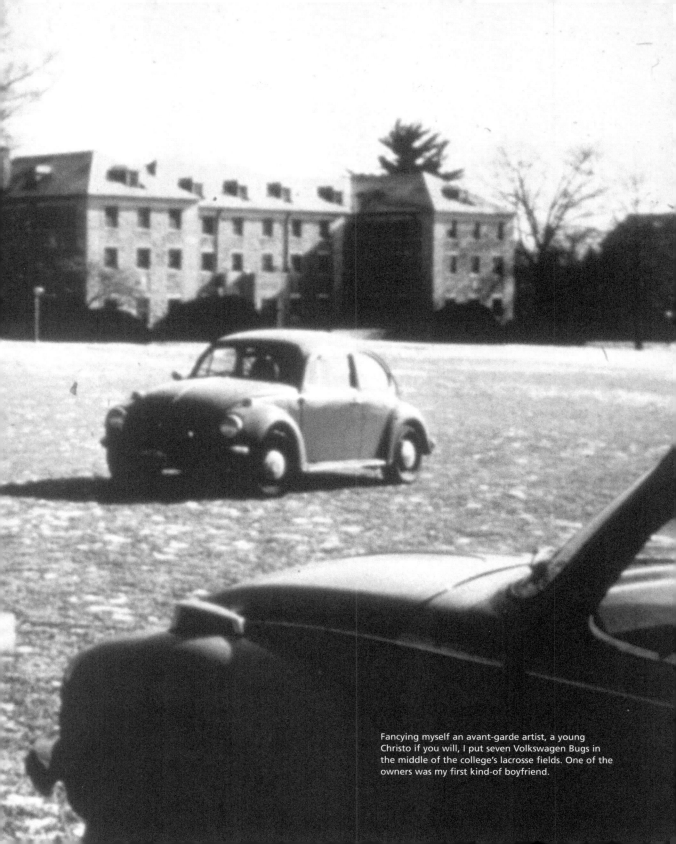

Fancying myself an avant-garde artist, a young Christo if you will, I put seven Volkswagen Bugs in the middle of the college's lacrosse fields. One of the owners was my first kind-of boyfriend.

After dinner, my now almost-more-than-a-friend friend and I went for a drive in his Bug. With nowhere to go, we drove to the Crystal Mall, one town over. As we pulled into the desolate parking lot, Dylan calmly told me that his dad had cancer. That he was dying. I didn't know what to say. I wanted to give him so much love. On the way back to school, stopped at a red light, I leaned over and kissed him in an effort to seem taken over by my passion for him. I wasn't dying to kiss him, but I was dying to want to kiss him because I wanted him to know that I liked him a lot, and that his skin wouldn't do anything to change my attraction to him, even though it did. I also wanted to distract him from the pain of losing his dad. And finally, I poured my tongue into his mouth because I wanted the type of romantic relationship where I passionately kissed my boyfriend at red lights, particularly red lights that overlooked an old-fashioned train station and the Long Island Sound.

Dylan lived in Abbey House—the co-op "alternative" dorm just across the street from campus, where there were more philosophy, history, and art students per dorm capita. The look at Abbey House was decidedly anti–college sweatshirt, and I felt very grown up semi-seeing someone who lived there.

One night, when Dylan and I were spooning on his double mattress on the floor, I felt the pressure against my butt that I knew I'd inevitably feel. Up until that point, I'd managed to just lie there as he cuddled me to sleep (which is not to say I wasn't plagued by my lack of interest in doing stuff with him as I wondered why it was so much easier for me to let the Eye-Flutterer do stuff than Dylan). That night, however, I decided, what with him and his body so obviously longing to be "loved," I should just get on with it. I didn't want to lose Dylan just because I didn't want to touch his thing.

Holding my breath, with my back still facing him, my right hand reached around and found its way down the front of his boxers. This was the awkward position from which I managed to "get him off." As I rubbed and rubbed, I wished that rubbing such a weird, not remotely attractive appendage wasn't such a prerequisite for continuing to date someone. Why did having such a great time with a guy mean I should be interested in touching his penis? I was relieved when my wondering and rubbing was finally interrupted by soft groans and wet stuff. Relaxed and ready to give me some sexual attention, Dylan started to kiss me as I tensed up. On a dime, I was able to escape into the refuge of sleep. Fear can be a surprisingly strong sleeping pill. I woke up the next morning, relieved that, as his semi-girlfriend, I had performed one of the "girlfriend things" I thought I should.

Getting a hand job from his semi-girlfriend was rare for poor Dylan. I somehow managed to continue to have a remarkable number of sleepovers where we didn't "do anything." I was racked with guilt at my lack of desire to touch him. I had desire—desire to hang out and talk and be silly. Just not to kiss and put my hands down his pants. He seemed to know I wasn't up for it and actually cared about me enough to not try to start something even though he clearly wanted to. I still desperately wanted to be the girlfriend that I had always envisioned I would be and that I was sure he hoped I would be. *Please, God, let me like sex*, I'd pray, even though I wasn't prone to prayer. *Please let there not be something wrong with my interest in sex. Please let me be normal.*

Very early one morning, the phone at Abbey House rang, so we both thought the same thing at the same time. Dylan had to go home again. This time, of course, for the funeral. Who knows what I must have said to a man who had just heard his father had died, but I was there for him and happy to be. While he was away, he let me drive his Bug. Downshifting up the campus drive, I distinctly felt very girlfriend. Our distance made it easier to embrace my new role.

And then, in an instant, school was over, and I was surprised I felt so ready and so relieved to be leaving Dylan. I flew back to L.A. to sell clothes at a boutique so I could earn some more money for my trip to Europe later in the summer. Dylan, on the other hand, had a life to create. He had to find a place to live and a place to work, and he had to attend to his newly widowed mother. He wrote me letters constantly. While I loved reading them and was flattered by the attention, I was also grateful he was three thousand miles away. Several letters later, he found the nerve to address the issue that had so plagued me and apparently him:

> My feelings for you then were not simply a love of admiration, infatuation, or yearning. You didn't fill any identifiable gap in my life like some relationships have and that took me by surprise. The sexual aspect of our experience was not central, like it becomes with some, and that was xpxkxxlxdx different

Before settling on the more diplomatic and nondescriptive "different," Dylan had written something else—more than likely something more descriptive and perhaps more wounding—that he then backspaced over with lots of other letters making the initial word unreadable. Desperate to know what he really thought, I held the letter up to the light. I turned it over. I studied it hard. But I couldn't figure out what he'd written. How did he really feel that the sexual aspect of our relationship wasn't "central"? I couldn't muster the nerve to ask—even in a letter.

He continued:

> The most beautiful part of our shared love was the mysterious strength you fed me while my father lay dying. I didn't feel as if you really knew what you were doing, but your clandestine support held me together in an honest way. I am filled w/a pang for what I think you to be. We have never really talked about things seriously. And I don't know why.

Well, I knew why. I had absolutely no idea how to begin to tell amazing, cool, fun, smart, caring, sensitive Dylan that I didn't want to "be in a relationship" with him because I wasn't attracted to him but that I wished I was because then I could continue to hang out with him without feeling like I was leading him on, without feeling the pressure to do stuff that I was ashamed to not want to do. *Why*, I vaguely wondered, *couldn't I be attracted to the guys I liked spending time with most?*, oblivious to the idea that there could actually be an answer to my question.

Not surprisingly, Dylan's sentiments were virtually identical to those Derek had written me in high school:

Derek: A lot has happened. We don't talk about it. I wonder why.

Dylan: We have never really talked about things seriously. And I don't know why.

And now the tables had turned. I was them, and John was me. *What more could I have wanted from Dylan?* I wondered, hoping an answer would help me be a better girlfriend to John. I guess what I would've wanted was reassurance that Dylan would have continued to love me and hug me and be with me, even though I didn't want to rub his penis or have sex. My fear was a fear of being left because of how I really felt. I certainly would understand Dylan not wanting a girlfriend who wasn't physically attracted to him, which is why I didn't want to tell him I wasn't. I loved being loved by him too much to lose him. *Was John feeling feelings similar to any of those feelings?*

six

scheduling sex

I was surprised that Neutral Patti wasn't recommending that John and I share our feelings with each other. Instead, she was recommending action. By session seven Neutral P. suggested that John and I schedule sex as a way to jump-start our intimacy. **SCHEDULING SEX** was what our life had come to. But it made sense the way Neutral P. had put it. If we scheduled it, then we wouldn't have it hanging over us every night. I wouldn't be lying in bed waiting for him to touch me, only to turn over simmering with rage that he hadn't, and John wouldn't have to feel the constant pressure to touch me that was clearly a total turnoff. Being good patients with the desire to be better partners to each other, we were willing to give this mortifying **SCHEDULING SEX** thing a try.

N.P. said that we didn't have to actually have sex the first time. She suggested perhaps a massage, something more sensual that would bring us closer. We could have sex after the massage . . . if we felt like it.

Had we ever given each other massages before—sensual massages? N.P. asked.

My first thought was, *Kill me that I'm sitting in a Beverly Hills therapist's office being asked if my boyfriend and I have ever given each other sensual massages before.* Then came the anger because the answer was no. No, we hadn't given each other sensual massages before. Massages, yes, but sensual ones that led to fucking—which is what I was assuming she meant by "sensual"—no.

And then I knew something for sure. I knew that leaving the decision of whether or not to have sex after the **SCHEDULED SENSUAL MASSAGE** was asking for trouble. We might have a nice time with this **SSM** stuff—God forbid—and then problems might arise when one did want to fuck—guess who?—and one didn't.

"Maybe we should only do the sensual massage part," I pragmatically offered, and N.P. agreed. *Why did I even have to point that out? I thought. Can't she see it's obvious that the option to have sex after the massage should not be left up in the air? Isn't the whole point of the exercise to not apply pressure? Why is she alleviating pressure only to reapply it?* I wanted a more competent therapist!

Neutral P. suggested we make our bedroom very romantic. She recommended using candles and silky scarves. And then she laughed because we looked at her like she was crazy. John and I were not scarf people. Couldn't she tell? What the fuck would we do with silk scarves? I envisioned an aqua scarf lying on the bed next to a naked me, with a naked John hovering over me. It not only didn't seem plausible, it seemed totally ridiculous. "I know that it might sound corny, but setting a mood can be really helpful," Patti explained. We agreed to candles, but scarves were out.

All week, John and I would say things to each other like, "Honey, just two more days until our **SCHEDULED SENSUAL MASSAGE**. I can't wait, sweetheart." Making fun of ourselves was all we could do to not plummet further into a depression.

Earlier in the day of our **SSM** night, I had gone out and bought a bottle of seventeen-dollar massage oil. Then, early the evening of, we just so happened to get into a fight—the cause of which I can't remember because it was of no significance. Being good therapy patients, we both figured we were probably just trying to sabotage our **SSM** even though there wouldn't even be any sex! How could we give each other sensual massages if we were too angry to even look at each other? To our credit, we managed to work our way through things enough to show up for our appointment. We were only an hour late.

I went into the kitchen and took all the candles we owned out of the cupboard. Votives, round, silver, and copper ones—leftover gifts from the holidays—and a bunch of tea-light candles. We placed them all around our bedroom, lit the wicks, and turned off the lights. Too bright! John blew some out while I went to the bathroom to get the expensive massage oil that he was touched I'd made a special effort to buy for the occasion. Then we flipped for it. Theoretically, I won because he would get his **SSM** first, which meant that after mine, I could continue to relax.

I was fairly confident that I gave good massages. And I did give him a good one, but did I give him a sensual one? I worked the oil deeply into his muscles in long hard strokes that I alternated with shorter ones. I flipped him over. I deeply massaged his inner thighs. I pulled his legs out from his ankles. And while I certainly worked hard, I didn't get him remotely hard. Perhaps it was because for John, lying naked is the equivalent of lying fully dressed, except that he's simply more comfortable. I was relaxing him but not exciting him. I wanted to excite him even though the point wasn't to excite him. My turn.

First he did my backside and then, like me, he flipped me over. But unlike him, I felt exposed and vulnerable. I wished my body just irresistibly and uncontrollably made him want to kiss me, touch me, and hold me tight. Maybe it did—and he was just following the no-sex **SSM** rules.

Afterward we briefly discussed how it had all gone.

"It really felt great, honey," he said, then adding that "it wasn't so sensual."

Hurt, I asked, "So is that why you didn't give me a sensual massage either? I mean you didn't even get anywhere near my area."

"Honey, I just didn't want to get any of that oil on your pubic hair," John explained.

"Well, I don't think it would've hurt me," I told him.

Oh God, I thought. Is *this really, could this possibly be, my life*? The answer being, "of course." Of course it's my life. I shouldn't have been so surprised. When had my sex life not been a surprise to me?

seven

nobody told me
there would be days like these

I distinctly remember the day, during my sophomore year of college, when my what-I-wouldn't-ever-have-wanted-it-to-be-like sex life became my what-I-never-ever-dreamed-it-would-include sex life. Most certainly, nobody told me there would be a day like that. A strange day indeed.

At nineteen years old, I was totally unprepared for the thoughts that flooded my brain that Christmas-break day I found myself getting up from my bath and humping the side of the porcelain tub. Sure, I'd heard masturbation was normal. But that's about all I'd heard. It's normal. It's normal. It's normal. *But how did it work*? I'd wondered. I mean, again thanks to *Fast Times at Ridgemont High*, I knew guys rubbed their penises to fantasies of hot women taking off their clothes, but what about us girls? Well, now I knew—kind of.

I was taking a two-week modern-dance intensive in New York City—staying at a friend's friend's studio—when it happened. After a day of exhausting classes and freezing weather, I took a bath while my friend and her friend hung out in the living/bed/only room watching TV. As I lay in the tub, no one was more surprised than I that my mind took me back to the veranda of the Miknos's Greek-island home, with the James-Bond-movie-worthy views of the Aegean that I'd visited that past summer at my college friend Miknos's invitation.

Miknos—yet another of my heavyset admirers—and I had hung out fairly often my freshman/his sophomore year. He was the only person I knew who smoked more than I did. I loved staying up real late, having conversations that were different from the ones I had with American guys. One late smoking night, I made the mistake of lying down on his bed. Despite finding him objectively unattractive, it wasn't too long before those please-I'm-begging-you-relieve-me-of-the-throbbing-between-my-legs feelings vied for my permission. As I struggled to think straight, I somehow managed to force myself to sit the fuck up and make my getaway, before I started something I didn't want to finish. I was careful to not put myself back in that Pete-type position again—but not careful enough, seeing that I accepted an invitation to visit him in Greece that upcoming summer.

Miknos was fat, just as Derek and Mickey had been. Their fat made them safe lovers for me.

The invitation to spend some time on a Greek island—just like Daryl Hannah did in that ménage à trois movie she was in with the guy from the *Idol Maker* that had riveted me as an eighth-grader—was so tantalizing that I knew I had to figure out a way to convince my parents to not only let me go, but also to help fund it. I presented the invitation as a once-in-a-lifetime opportunity for an adventure. (Wasn't part of the allure of sending me to an East Coast college to expand my horizons? To meet different kinds of people?) I told them I'd work at a summer job to make some of the money, and that I'd be traveling with my girlfriend from school. A few months later, I found myself on a transatlantic flight with my stick-in-the-mud friend who I didn't yet know was a stick-in-the-mud.

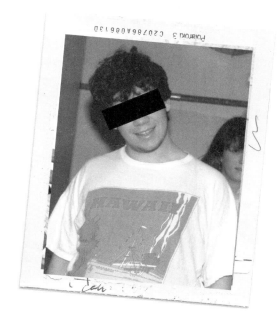

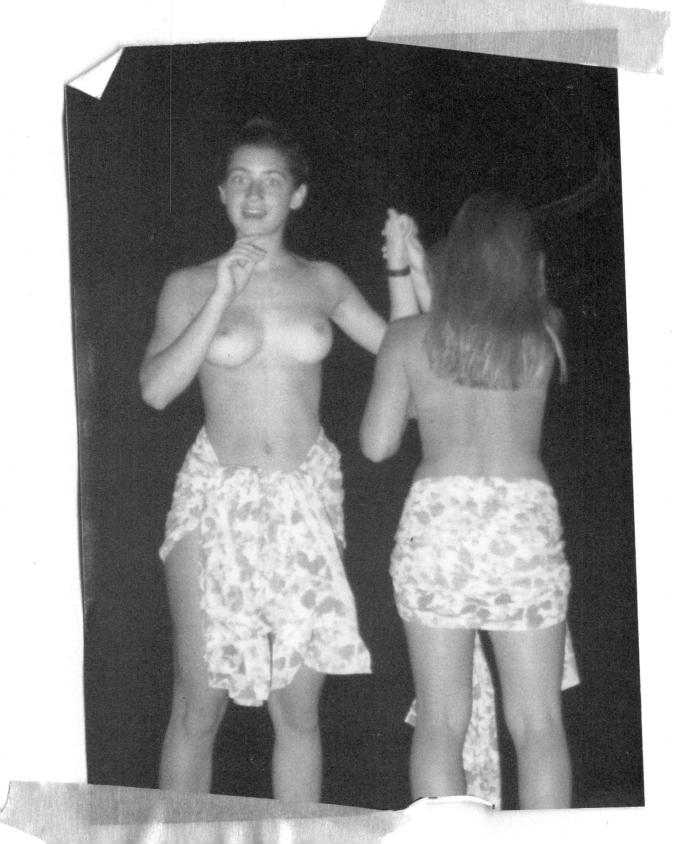

Miknos was the perfect host. He wined and dined us. He bought us tickets to the ballet at the Acropolis. And during our weeklong stay at his old family home on the magnificent island of Sífnos, he gave us a thorough tour, took us out to the nightclubs, and was a gentleman—meaning he didn't make a move on me throughout the entire trip, until, of course, the last night when we were back at his parents' home in Athens. The stick-in-the-mud was asleep in the other room when Miknos told me that our trip to Sífnos was his first ever with a girl that he didn't have sex with. I guess his way of seducing me was to tell me how nice he had been all week by not trying to seduce me. Or maybe he was trying to seduce me by making me feel like I owed him something, like I wasn't living up to the unspoken part of the bargain. Or maybe he was saying how usually women are just so overcome by the beauty of the island that sex just happens. Or maybe he was saying how prudish we Americans are. Or maybe he was saying he felt like a loser in front of his friends because he couldn't get the American girl who he'd told them had come all this way to be with him. Whatever he was saying by saying something else, it worked, because I leaned over and kissed him, which he took to mean, "Let's fuck."

It happened so quickly. And, unfortunately, it happened with the lights on, so I only had my eyelids to hide his frenzied fat body and his disconcerting, uncircumcised penis from view. But, for some reason, I was incredibly curious about the goings-on and watched as if it wasn't me that stuff was being done to. I watched him take my underwear off and dive between my legs, only to emerge seconds later to pull a pubic hair out of his mouth as if that was a normal thing to do. Then he asked me to sit on his face— something I'd not only never done nor been asked to do, but something I'd never heard of. So I straddled his face as he went at it—doing what, I'm not exactly sure—as I braced myself by palming the wall just millimeters in front of my nose. Finally, it was time for him to screw me. He flipped me on my back, donned a condom, and pummeled away. As soon as he came, he apologized for not doing a better job. "I'm sorry. It's just that I was so excited," he said. "Do you want some yogurt with honey?"

Me and my stick-in-the-mud friend on Miknos's veranda on the island of Sífnos. Prancing around in next to nothing, we craved the attention of Miknos and his friends, but had no intention of satisfying the desire that we undoubtedly stirred in them.

I nodded yes as he leaped out of bed and ran down to the kitchen to prepare me the very Greek snack. Eating it was the best part of the night.

But that auspicious day in that New York tub, my mind wasn't referencing Miknos and his Greek friends alone. Out of nowhere, my subconscious was drawing from this long-forgotten trashy novel I'd happened upon during my fifteen-turning-sixteen summer. I don't remember the title or the plot—only this one memorable scene starring a very beautiful, tall, tan, thin woman with a pixie haircut who was trapped in a weird/abusive relationship with a big slimy man whose friends (mobsters/pigs) were always around.

My trashy-novel-meets-Greek-island fantasy, which got me so worked up that I felt compelled to hump the side of the tub, went something like this:

Miknos was the man and I, of course, was the woman and the friends (mobsters) pigs were Miknos's friends—Adonis, Alessandro, and Christos. Miknos greeted his cohorts with hugs, kisses, and Greek words of welcome as everyone took a seat. Then I, naked, went from man to man, sitting on their laps, my legs straddled around their bellies. Each would fondle me until Miknos nodded his head, indicating that he should let me go so I could move on to the next guy. No one could do more to me than Miknos would allow. The weird part is that everyone knew I was Miknos's special friend and that in other circumstances we all hung out normally, but that I also did this type of stuff for Miknos. It was a privilege that Miknos let them touch me. Over time, I'd come to envision them all in the bedroom, smoking cigarettes and drinking scotch as they each took turns staring at or actually licking my "down there."

Soon after I started to get off via fantasies of being objectified by Miknos and then fucking the side of the tub, driven by the pain of my continuously bruised pelvic bone, I discovered the faucet. If I positioned myself just so, got the water at just the right pressure and at just the right lukewarm temperature, I could come just as easily—though perhaps not quite as hard. Another option, I soon discovered, was that right at the I-just-can't-take-it-anymore point, I'd tell myself to get out of tub and lie facedown on my bed—which would prolong the pleasure that much longer—and then I'd hump the certainly-softer-than-porcelain mattress. When I saw Madonna do the same thing in her slow rendition of "Like a Virgin" in her *Blond Ambition* documentary, I was relieved to learn that she sometimes got off by fucking the bed, too! *Was she breaking ground or was it common knowledge that women got off that way?* I wondered.

I was curious about masturbation. Why did I think these thoughts? Why/how did they get me so worked up? Why was getting off by conjuring up weird fantasies of being objectified by European chauvinists so much easier than getting excited by "making love" with a real, live, loving, caring guy like Dylan? And, finally, what did getting off have to do with love? I'd heard from friends that when you had sex with someone you truly loved, it was so different, so much better. But how was it?

To make matters even more confusing to an undergraduate me, I was starting to think of myself as a feminist—a word and idea I'd never heard of before college. My new best friend, Katie, was my teacher. We were women, she told me. Not girls. And we were people, not sex objects. We were to be respected, not degraded. She really drove the point home when we heard about this crudely made dummy a bunch of students found in the fields next to the arboretum.

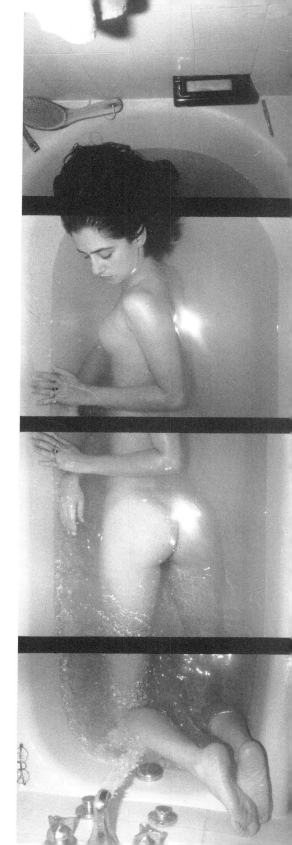

Me in my new favorite place. I didn't know why I thought the thoughts I thought, but I couldn't help thinking them.

Rumor had it that the rugby team had been at it again. Just like the year before, as part of their initiation for new players, they made a stuffed figure, dressed it in a skirt and bra, smeared cottage cheese all over its thighs, and placed a can of tuna between the stumps that passed as legs. Apparently, this lovely creation was for the new recruits to faux-fuck. It was tradition.

Well, Katie was outraged. And so was I! What could degrading women possibly have to do with trying to get a ball into a goal? The more we fumed about it, the madder we got, which led to an idea. Katie and I marched over to my dorm room, sat down at the computer, and wrote a letter that we addressed to the president of the college, to all of the deans, and to the entire faculty and administration. We were aghast over the apparent acceptance of this representation of women, as evidenced by the lack of action after the figure was reported. And surely, the coach of the team knew about this behavior and did nothing to discourage it. We edited it and rewrote it and edited it and rewrote it until it was perfectly sound, defiant, and outraged. And then we made hundreds of copies and headed over to the post office.

The team was suspended for the year. The incident was reported in the *College Voice* and the ritual was deleted from the team's annual activities. We couldn't believe it. And neither could the players and their coach. While I'm sure they wanted to kill us, they weren't privy to our names. All of the other teams took notice—we hoped. While we were glad they were suspended, we wondered if they had been educated.

The more informed I became, the more confused I was. Why did I, someone who condemned the objectification of women, need to fantasize about being objectified in order to attend to the desire inside of me that I could no longer ignore? These were strange, hard-to-make-sense-of days indeed.

eight

objectifying

One rare occasion when John and I were in bed with our clothes off, and I was on top passionately doing something—kissing, bucking, writhing—John did the worst thing I could imagine. He laughed. Angry that he was not only not mirroring my passion, but that he was making fun of it, I asked him what was so fucking funny.

"Honey, I'm not laughing at you. It's just that you're sooo melodramatic. I'm just enjoying you."

"Enjoying me? What do you mean? I feel like you think I'm a joke. I want to be found hot or erotic while I'm fucking, not funny."

"It's not so much that I think you're funny, honey. It's just amazing how you get so totally into it. It's like you're on your own. You're not finding what's between us. I think we should try to find what's between us."

I'd heard it before from John. He felt like I was forcing my sex agenda on him, regardless of how he was feeling. I just didn't know what he meant by "finding what's between us." What was between us and how were we supposed to find it? What would sex be like when we found what was between us? To escape our discomfort at a conversation that we didn't know where to take, we turned on the TV.

Lying there, I had sense enough to remind myself that it was probably a good thing that John didn't just get off because he loved my breasts (which he did), or the very sight of my pussy, because apparently, given my track record, and gleaning from Neutral P.'s fear-of-intimacy diagnosis, I needed to learn about real love and intimacy. *What*, I wondered, *is the difference between getting aroused by finding a body beautiful and getting off by objectifying someone's body?*

And to be honest, I wasn't getting off just because I found John's body beautiful, though I did find it incredibly beautiful. I was totally in my head, almost using John's body—which he must've detected. Screwing him, I was busy fantasizing about something I'd never have the courage to share with John or Neutral Patti. John's laughter interrupted my fantasy of being a prostitute who was screwing a paralyzed vet who just so happened to look like John (and not like Tom Cruise in *Born on the 4th of July*). What could be less intimate?

John was right. We had to find what was between us.

nine

the captain of wonkville

Despite the honors and distinction on my diploma, I didn't get the college education I desperately needed. More than my classes on Kant, Hinduism, statistics, choreography, Islamic art, or anthropology, what I needed—even though I had absolutely no idea I needed it—was a class on attraction, sexuality, and communication. Relationships 101 should have been a prerequisite. What course could possibly have a greater impact on a student's entire life and ultimately his/her offspring?

So, unarmed with the education I needed, I went out into the world searching for both love and a life.

I decided to forgo the safety of graduate school and just go for living in New York. Fortunately, I found a great East Village tenement apartment, lucked into the perfect roommate, and landed the $7.50-an-hour part-time job doing computer work at a dance studio that I had to campaign for as if it was a position that could ever lead to anything better. Soon after my roommate and I bought identical black motorcycle boots on St. Marks Place, I felt

Despite the honors and distinction on my diploma, I didn't get the education I desperately needed. Relationships 101 wasn't in the course catalog.

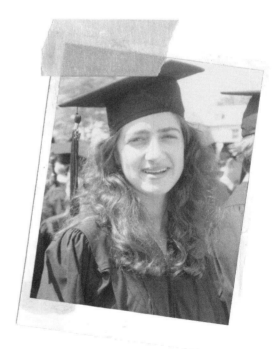

ready to embark on my life as an artist in earnest. Needless to say, my parents were still paying for my rent, my health insurance, my plane tickets, and other sundry bills.

It was at my feminist heroine friend Katie's birthday party that I met Auggie—a beautiful olive-skinned guy with the most Venus-flytrap eyelashes I'd ever seen. Though a year older than me, Auggie was finishing up his undergrad degree in photography and working part-time at a charming bookstore in the West Village.

Even though our conversation was very "How do you know Katie?," I could tell right away that not only was he extraordinarily beautiful, Auggie was sweet, gentle, and smart—though a bit shy. For once, there was nothing not to be attracted to.

After our first romantic dinner date, I managed to hide the orgasm that passed through me as we made out on my bed. As usual, the second it had, the desire for contact instantly drained from my body and I wanted to stop making out, which was perfect for a first date because it made me seem not so easy.

Unfortunately for both of us, I never again felt so turned on with Auggie. I loved being affectionate, holding hands and kissing, but it didn't get me worked up. There I was, loving my new perfect boyfriend, dreading his overtures. Confused by my lack of interest and in a feeble effort to broach the uncomfortable subject, Auggie told me how much his last girlfriend absolutely loved sex. I couldn't think of anything to say as I thought I wanted nothing more than to be her.

My response wasn't to share my feelings. It was to have sex. I wouldn't let more than a month go by without screwing. I instinctually felt that that was about as long as I could push it without us having to verbally acknowledge that we had a problem and that the problem was me. In the meantime, I gave him blow jobs in an attempt to appease him, to disguise the fact that we weren't doing it. Do you think he noticed?

It was during these blow jobs that I actually came to love Auggie's penis. His was the first penis I befriended—the first one that I personified. With all of the experiences that I'd had, I'd managed to rarely see any guy's penis until it was time for me to hold it or rub it or suck it. And that I could do with my eyes closed or in the dark. Penises were ugly and weird. But then I got to know my new friend, Captain Wonk, the Mayor of Wonkville, and felt differently.

I was relieved to have a level of comfort with Auggie that enabled me to get the anatomy lesson that I needed. I was finally able to sit still and take it all in—what a flaccid penis looked and felt like, how hairs sprouted out of the shriveled-up scrotal skin, what the veins on the shaft looked like, and perhaps most interestingly, how his stuff actually connected to the rest of his body. And I had no idea that a guy's area could smell so sweet! I loved sniffing him. After I had christened his "wonk" Captain Wonk, the Mayor of Wonkville, I named his balls Deputy One and Deputy Two—though like two identical twins, I didn't really know which was which.

It wasn't unusual for us to be lying in bed when I'd peel off his boxers and scoot myself down for a visit. While I gently kissed and touched him I'd croon, "Hi there, Captain. Oh, you sure do smell good today. Did you know I've missed you Won-kee? I've missed you soooo much."

Auggie seemed to enjoy the friendship I was building with the Captain

I could not have found a more beautiful, gentle, and smart boyfriend. I loved to look at him and touch him— just not to have sex with him. Sound familiar?

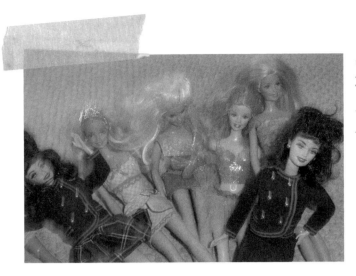

My relationship to Auggie's penis and balls—which I affectionately referred to as "The Mayor of Wonkville and his Deputies"—was similar to the relationship a girl might have with her Barbies.

and his deputies. Perhaps he was happy to have any type of sexual attention—though I don't know if you could classify my talking to and fondling his stuff as if they were Barbie dolls as sexual. Maybe he was just happy to have the attention period.

Despite the sexual awkwardness of our relationship, we created a nice life for ourselves. We alternated between my apartment and his industrial loft in the financial district. We went to dinner, to the movies, and out for drinks with friends—which meant either with my roommate or his. I worked on my art/art career and he printed his photographs. Not a lot of fanfare, just two young artists who found comfort in each other in the big, scary city.

Meanwhile, my artwork was starting to make its way into the world. An installation I'd proposed was accepted by the New Museum of Contemporary Art to be a part of a (bad) exhibition. Soon thereafter, the Volkswagen Bug project that I was still peddling was accepted by the Cleveland Performance Art Festival. I had even received a personally written note from the director of the Walker Art Center inquiring about my work. The interest helped me show my parents that I was for real—that their monthly rent checks were paying off—kind of. Of course these invitations weren't bringing in money. On the contrary, I needed money to create the work.

Thanks to my great-aunt who died, I had an account with some sixteen thousand dollars that I wasn't supposed to touch, but continually siphoned from. My mother, who got the statements, surely knew but didn't say a word. She did mention, however, that my frequent calls home were getting very expensive. *What*?! I thought. *Doesn't she want to hear from me? Isn't she not-remotely poor? Didn't she wonder if a child who was calling home a lot was lonely?* I thought my mother was communicating her anxiety over my career choice, poor-excuse-for-an-income, and expensive place of residence by talking about the high phone bills I was costing her (without mentioning the rent, plane fares, insurances, etc. that she was covering). I was fairly confident that I knew what she was saying by saying something else, even if she didn't.

I also didn't appreciate the phone call where my mother said that her best friend had a nice (read: Jewish) guy to set me up with. "Mother, I have a boyfriend, as you well know!" I exclaimed, furious that she clearly had no respect for my relationship. She'd never asked about Auggie or how we were doing and now I knew why.

"Well, honey, it never hurts to explore your options," was her response.

Did she think that, at twenty-two, I was remotely close to even thinking about marriage and contemplating how I wanted to raise my children?

A year later, our still super-erratic and unfulfilling sex life was wearing on poor Auggie. It seemed that my tide-him-over blow jobs weren't enough. Without knowing the right way to broach the subject, he uncharacteristically told me a joke.

"How does a Jewish girl eat a banana?" he asked one Sunday morning as we were walking out of a bodega, having just purchased a newspaper and cigarettes.

"I don't know," said I, the Jewish girl.

Pretending to hold a banana in his left hand, he "unpeeled" it with his right hand. Then he placed his right hand on the back part of his head and pushed it down toward the banana—faux-forcing himself to eat it.

I was hurt, but at least the ice was finally broken. We couldn't just ignore the fact that I never wanted to screw forever.

"Jennifer," he said, "I don't know what the problem is. I can only think that you might be, well, I think you might be frigid."

Frigid? Was that really a condition one had? I wondered. If I have it, is it something I might have forever? Could I be frigid but still get off in the tub to visions of being served to Vas on a tray at a party, as if my vagina was an appetizer to enjoy before the main course?

So the next time Auggie and I were hanging out and I actually felt somewhat interested in having him do stuff to me, I thought it behooved me to share the sexual thoughts flashing through my mind. We were sitting in my living room when I got up the nerve to whisper in his ear how I wanted to be on all fours while he touched me. Saying the words out loud turned me on even more. He was happy I was up for some sex stuff. I told him to wait just a moment, I had to go to the bathroom first.

So I went. And out of nowhere I had diarrhea. Fuck, why now?!?! Why now, when I'm finally feeling like I want to fuck my boyfriend who is sick and tired of me not fucking him? It was a mess. It wasn't totally liquid diarrhea, it was more sludgish. I tried to clean myself up as quickly as I possibly could because I didn't want these rare sexual feelings to pass me by. I didn't want to disappoint Auggie.

Somehow, the emphasis on *how*, I must've wiped some shit from the back part to the front part. And I didn't get it all. And I thought I had. I thought I had done a good job of cleaning up the mess. How could a 22-year-old girl not know if she was or was not doing a good job wiping herself?! How?!

So I joined him in my bedroom and lay down. Auggie, unaware of the explosion, lifted my skirt and took off my underpants. And then he went down there to lick me and he saw the traces of shit on my vagina. Quietly and gently he said, "You need to go back to the bathroom."

Needless to say, I wanted to kill myself.

ten

another appointment

At our Tuesday appointment following our **SCHEDULED SENSUAL MASSAGE**, Neutral Patti was pleased to hear that we'd followed through with the assignment. I didn't say a word about how not so sensual it really was. Neither did John. Our omission must've given Neutral P. the wrong impression, because she gave us our next assignment: **TO SCHEDULE SEX**! Instantly nervous that the scheduling would loom over us all week long—me not mentioning it, afraid of applying pressure, and John avoiding it—I tried to discreetly suggest that it might be better to schedule our appointment right then and there. N.P. got the message and asked us when we thought might be a good time.

John got his calendar out of his backpack, flipped to the week in question and offered Friday at seven-thirty. Done.

Friday at seven-thirty we both showed up right on time. Because our assignment didn't include a sensual massage before the sex, we just went ahead and got right to it. In my head I lamented the lack of foreplay but didn't say a word. At the same time I was just relieved that his penis was actually inside my vagina—feelings reminiscent of a sixteen-year-old-virgin me, mortified by my embarrassing condition, relieved to finally be able to say I had done it. And I did come. And so did he. So what was the problem, right? Well, for me, coming wasn't necessarily the sign of a successful screw. All I had to do to come was have my ass cheeks spread apart a little (which John knew), or think some dirty thought, and then boom—orgasm. I could come on a dime. But I longed for something more. I wanted John to be more into me.

Back at N.P.'s for our next Tuesday session, I opened with a less than enthusiastic report about our **SCHEDULED SEX NIGHT.** And while I thought I was doing what we were supposed to be doing in therapy—telling the truth—I didn't realize how much I was hurting John. Here he'd complied with the assignment. We'd had sex. I had an orgasm. What the fuck else did I want from him? Here was more proof that I was insatiable—a bottomless pit that would never get enough or the right kind of kisses or hugs or sex for my liking.

N.P. had to agree. I had an overwhelming tendency to see the glass as half empty. I should have been happy we had had sex after not having done it for so long. I should've been grateful that my boyfriend was so willing to work on this stuff, both in therapy and at home.

Wow, I thought, I *really am a glass-half-emptier*. I felt terrible and so did John. I was sure my glass-half-empty attitude would set us back some. I mean, who would want to screw someone so fucking critical and insatiable? I'd really fucked up this time. And who did I blame? My poor mother. She wasn't known for her glass-half-full outlook on life and now I was becoming her! I couldn't believe it was true. Glass-half-empty meant you were pessimistic because you were afraid of being optimistic. Glass-half-empty was synonomous with FEAR.

eleven

finally

It had been over a decade since my parents had sold their private elementary school to devote themselves entirely to their art business. My Dad was the art dealer (visionary, aesthete, salesmen, all-around debonair guy) and my mother was the behind-the-scenes-do-everything-elser (bookkeeper, taxpayer, office organizer, letter writer, insurance arranger, all-around hard worker). They were both well suited for their positions, but only one had the stomach for the business.

My father was a risk taker by nature who had a certain faith that he'd be successful. My mother, on the other hand, couldn't get over the fact that they were (she was) putting their livelihoods in the hands of "well-to-do" people who might or might not be in the mood to buy art. As hard as she worked, as many numbers as she crunched, as perfectly as she balanced the checkbook, their income was out of her control. There always remained the distinct possibility—and perhaps, realistically, the likelihood—that she might not be rewarded for her stay-up-until-three-in-the-morning efforts. Creating innovative school programs, such as library skills and sex education, was a lot more fulfilling for her, but after twenty years, my dad had had it with running a school. He had a new life to lead, and my mom wanted him to be happy. So she followed his lead.

And now my dad was mounting his most ambitious and most expensive project to date—a massive outdoor sculpture exhibition along the coast. He would be installing works up to twenty-five feet high, weighing up to several tons, on the beach, on lawns, in fields, in shopping centers, in restaurants, and even in parking lots. The endless stream of bills for the crates, the flatbed trucks, the shipping, the installation, the insurance, the cranes, the printing, and the advertising was, well, never-ending. It was a dream-come-true project for my father, and a living nightmare for my mother.

My parents desperately needed my self-taught graphic-design and public-relations skills, which had been honed by years of writing grants, cover letters, applications and résumés, and designing press kits for me and all of my artist friends. And so, I left New York and Auggie for the summer to help my parents, who'd helped me in every way they could for my entire life.

Proud of my newly acquired Adobe Illustrator skills, I set out to create all of the literature for the exhibition. I was also my dad's sounding board. Having raised me to share my strong opinions on whether this painting looked better here or there, next to this sculpture or that plant, he appreciated my eye. I was happy to have my talents put to good use. It certainly beat a hot, muggy summer in New York entering numbers into Quicken at the dance studio.

And while the planning of the show was going smoothly, there was a great deal of tension around. And I always sided with my dad. Since they'd already committed to this exhibition, I couldn't understand why my mother kept getting so upset about the cost of everything. It was already in motion, so why not be optimistic about its success? What was agonizing over every single aspect of it going to do? But she just couldn't help herself. She was so afraid that this time my dad had risked too much, that the comfortable life they enjoyed was seriously at risk. So every time her fear would riddle him with guilt and anxiety, I'd try to cheer him up by telling him what an incredible job he was doing and how amazing it was going to be. I felt I had to bolster him and calm her, but sometimes I was too upset at her raining on his parade to be kind. Sometimes both my dad and I couldn't take my mother's lamenting anymore and we'd double-team my poor mother. But then, as if he wasn't behaving in the exact same way, my father would get mad at me for being so hard on my mother. She was doing her best and working so hard and was under a lot of strain. I should have more respect for her. It wasn't unusual for this pattern to repeat itself several times throughout the course of the week.

In addition to my (failed) attempts at mediation and my graphic-design work, I would also be working in the gallery and giving public tours of the exhibition to strangers in an airport minivan (a job I didn't like but was amazingly good at). And for all of this work, how would I be compensated? Well, that wasn't something we ever discussed.

I figured that my parents were so caught up in their emotions and the fast-approaching opening deadline, they didn't have time to consider it. After all, I was living at home and their housekeeper was making all of my meals, and they did fly me out and they had been paying my rent and various other bills for a long time/my whole fucking life. And I did have their gas card for gas, so what did I need money for? And while I agreed with that argument (that they never presented), I still needed some spending money. Sometimes my mom would give me fifty dollars and sometimes my dad would give me twenty, but there was no rhyme or reason to it. And the last thing I wanted to do was ask my mom for money, when here my dad was spending too much of it already.

Though Auggie and I were still officially together, it had been more than several months since I'd thought we should probably end things. While I still felt guilty that we weren't having the sex life he wanted, there were other problems. His behavior was starting to grate on me. It was more what he wasn't doing than what he was. He seemed to have a lack of ambition. He also could go an entire dinner party without once contributing to the conversation. Neither of us had yet begun to learn how to communicate, probably because we didn't know we didn't know how. Providing each other with a safe haven from a scary world wasn't enough. And so I wasn't entirely surprised that almost upon landing in Los Angeles, I felt a surge in my libido. There's nothing like getting three thousand miles away from your lover to make a frigid girl horny.

Immediately falling back into my old high school habits, one day while driving in Malibu, I stopped by Bobbie's family beach house with a friend of mine named Chivas—uninvited. Bobbie wasn't home, but his best friend was. I'd been attracted to the young Sam Shepardesque TJ ever since I'd met him a few years earlier. Instantly, I was overcome by desire. So while TJ and Chivas played chess next to the pool, I did my best to seduce.

I dove in in my underwear and soon-to-be see-through tank. I bobbed up and down, swam on my back, and occasionally got out, only to dive in again. And seduce I did. As soon as TJ won, he jumped in after me. Totally rude and absorbed in each other, we started kissing as if Chivas wasn't there. Ten or maybe even twenty-five minutes later, Chivas realized we weren't going to take a break anytime soon, so he left to get some sushi. Meanwhile, for the next two hours, with my legs tightly wrapped around TJ's waist, we sank down, pushed up, gasped for air, pushed off, drifted, and sank some more. By far, it was the most unforgettable, exciting, satisfying, sexy make-out of my life and still holds the record to this day, some ten years later. Unfortunately, getting naked on the beach twenty minutes later, uncomfortably fooling around in the sand and feeling pressure to fuck, sucked. But it didn't suck so much that I didn't want to be with him. On the contrary, I wanted to be with him even more. Any feelings of guilt about cheating on Auggie were completely obliterated by this blind desire to re-play that scene in the pool one more time. It was as if the after-scene on the beach had never happened.

When TJ invited me out for dinner the next week, I couldn't wait. What he had to tell me, however, came as a shock.

"I know you have a boyfriend, and think it's okay to 'hang out,' but I just don't feel comfortable doing that. I mean I think you're cool and all, but this just can't happen."

I couldn't believe what I was hearing. I couldn't understand how he could possibly not want to be with me after we'd experienced what we'd experienced. How could it matter that I hadn't officially broken up with Auggie yet? How could TJ want to continue living without making out in the pool like that again? (I didn't realize, of course, that the romp in the pool could never have been so intense had I been unattached.) The only thing that gave me solace was the fact that I wasn't frigid after all.

My rebound from TJ, however, became more than just a rebound. He was, in fact, a life alterer. A sex-life alterer. His name was Stuart, and he was an actor who was fairly new to Hollywood. We were introduced by a mutual friend one evening at a bar. By the end of the night, my number had been asked for and soon we were on the phone telling each other about our lives. I was impressed that, inspired by an experience in an acting class and encouraged by a mentor, he had decided to take an entirely different road. I respected a man who had left a safe life for an unsure, artistic one. I was looking forward to our dinner date.

As usual, I enjoyed the first-date seduction. It's when I always felt my most confident, charming, and witty. I liked talking about my artistic ventures, which I felt helped establish me as a smart, you'll-never-meet-anyone-else-like-me person. We ended the date whispering under the stars in the backyard of his aunt and uncle's house where he was staying (rent-free) until he could get on his feet. The tension to kiss was building beautifully and soon we were rolling around on the cement. As usual I quickly but silently came, which meant I was ready to go home.

Our second date ended on the floor of my parents' beach house, with me trying to focus on the pain of the rug burns on my knees as a way to help bring myself to orgasm. It didn't work, but I was surprised that I thought it might. I'd never contemplated pain as an aphrodisiac before. When our oh-so-sexy screw was over, we went to the balcony and looked at the ocean. In my his-oxford-with-no-underpants look, I liked how I hoped I looked. I didn't like how I felt, but was used to that.

So after my second date with Stuart—which he loved—I reluctantly told a suspicious Auggie that we were over. He was so sad. He sent me a birthday card in which he told me he loved me—it was the first time he'd done that in the almost two years we'd been dating. (I guess I wasn't the only one who had a fear of intimacy.) I felt terrible that I felt so vacant when I read the words. I hated having to hurt him, but I also wanted to date Stuart—which I did.

Our next few dates were similar in flavor. One of those nights we ended up fucking on the bathroom floor of the maid's room at his aunt and uncle's. More discomfort. More rug burns. No orgasm. But pride in how I thought I successfully came off as the adventurous, fun, sex-loving girl I wanted to be, because I thought that would not only be a fun person to be but a person who would continue to get the adoring love I was loving getting. Soon we were always either on the phone or in each other's arms. Every night we made out on the little bed in the maid's room for hours. I preferred the nights when we didn't fuck. We hated that I couldn't sleep over because of his aunt and uncle, so we pushed my departure time as long as we could—usually until three or four in the morning.

When Stuart got a house-sitting job, everything changed. He moved into a great place in the Hollywood Hills and basically I did, too. One day he was screwing me from behind when all of the sudden I felt his penis in the wrong place! It didn't go all the way in, just a little. And it hurt a little bit. And I was intrigued.

Hanging out at the beach the next day, I mustered the nerve to say, "I liked it when you did you-know-what yesterday."

"When I did what?"

"You know, when you went into the other place."

"Really?" he said, his eyes lighting up. "I didn't notice. But I like the sound of it."

We both did. We were excited. Excited to try it for real. Excited to have found someone to sexually experiment with!

Cut to me, on all fours, with Stuart behind—hyperaware of what we were trying to do. With no lubricant, Stuart ever so slowly guided his way in. I remember liking the combination of the pain of my asshole being split apart, the idea of how dirty I thought it was, and the increased pleasure that came when he reached around and rubbed my clitoris. After some steady rubbing and fucking, we both just couldn't take it another second and actually came simultaneously. We loved it. Finally, there I was—a girl who loved sex. Thank you, God. Thank you, Stuart.

Our kinkiness got kinkier. Soon I was out back in my little schoolgirl skirt leaning over the grill as he gently spanked me with his belt, only to then bring me inside, bend me over the bed, place the belt on the small of my back, and fuck me up the ass as I dug my pelvis into the mattress. Things were going from better to even better.

But after the novelty of the daring sex wore off a few weeks later, Stuart felt claustered by me. I was too needy. I wanted too much attention. Maybe I was on vacation from my life in New York, but he had a serious acting career to attend to. One night while he was busy watching TV in the living room, I walked in naked—pathetically hoping that at least sex might get his attention. He was busy with the commercials and couldn't be bothered. He didn't know how to say he needed space and I couldn't bear to give it. Standing there rejected in my birthday suit was the low point of the summer; despite that, I couldn't seem to stop myself from replicating the experience on several more occasions. My response to this rejection was always the same: I'd break down in tears, looking for attention, unable to express myself in any other way. My tears did nothing but drive Stuart even further away. I was too much to handle.

Soon, the end of the summer saved me from a cycle of rejection, tears, space, and sex, rejection, tears, space, and sex. I cried all the way to the airport, assuming Stuart was happy to have his summer fling leave town, which is why I was surprised by his frequent calls once I was back in New York. He said he missed me. Quite a lot, actually. He wanted to fly out to see me. Even though I sensed something awry inside me, I told him to come, sure, that sounded great. I mean, I had just spent my last week in L.A. in a constant state of wanting his attention, crying uncontrollably about leaving him. And didn't our new-kind-of-sex discovery give us a special bond? Why *wouldn't* I want him to come? I couldn't answer my own questions, so I gave him my address.

A few days later, my roommate, Pam, and I were hanging out in the living room waiting for Stuart to arrive. When he finally walked in the door, he looked completely different to me. In L.A., I thought his poofy, curly hair looked cool. In the East Village, it just looked goofy. His big toothy smile was too big and too toothy. Even his voice . . . I didn't want to hear it. I couldn't understand what had changed. All I definitively knew, without question, was that I was not remotely interested in or attracted to Stuart, and that I hated myself for getting into this very avoidable mess. I was relieved that Pam was there, so we could all chitchat while I figured out how to handle the bed I'd made and now had to lie in.

Eventually, we had no choice but to say good night to Pam and retire to my bedroom. I tried to be kind, but it was obvious: I wasn't into him being there, although I didn't have the nerve to say it. But he knew and said as much. Now that he'd spent all the money he didn't have flying across the country to be with the woman he finally realized he deeply loved, however, he felt I owed him a romantic night. Without thinking that if he truly loved me he wouldn't pressure me, I agreed with him. He told me I didn't have to do anything. He would just touch me and I could just relax and enjoy it. I agreed to the plan—not wanting him to feel more rejected than he already did. And wasn't that what I liked, being done to, not doing?

So I just lay there and let him fuck me. His hovering felt claustrophobic. His tongue felt sticky on my neck. What I had previously craved now repulsed me. Why, when I got what I thought I wanted, did I not want it anymore? That subconscious of mine was really working overtime.

The next morning it was clear that he should leave. As terrible as I felt for the position I'd put him in, I was relieved when he was gone—so relieved that I stopped contemplating the why of it all and just started back on my directionless, oblivious search for the right guy.

twelve

n.p.'s big idea

John told Neutral Patti that, during sex, he thought I was trying to control everything. Let's kiss this way, turn me over now, pin me down, spread me, spank me . . . whatever. He reiterated what he'd said many times before, which was that I didn't ever try to "find what was between us."

And he was right. I wasn't trying to find what was between us because I was busy trying to recapture what, at one point, had been between me and Stuart. Our sexual high had lasted a short time but made quite an impression. For a little while, it had brought Stuart and me closer together. And best of all, it had happened organically. But while we certainly had a sexual connection, it didn't translate into a healthy relationship. So I don't know why I was so busy trying to be with John in a way I'd been with Stuart. My attempts to control were only pushing us apart.

In response to John's complaint, Neutral Patti had an idea. For our next couple of **SCHEDULED SEX NIGHTS,** we were to alternate who would be in control of the sexing. That way I'd be forced to let things happen in a new way. We'd flip for who would be in charge first.

After hearing how much John didn't like my controlling the sex, I wanted him to win the toss, but of course he didn't and I did. But seeing that I was the patient and not the therapist, I was going to go ahead with Neutral P.'s plan.

So when the time of our **SCHEDULED SEX NIGHT** rolled around, we both showed up, disrobed, and hopped in bed. After some awkward attempts to get things going on my part, I leaned back and looked at John's face. He could not have been less into it. I felt like I was trying to make out with a blowup doll. His eyes were glazed over and he just lay there limp. He wasn't there. This was serious. Something was really wrong. "Honey," I said, "we don't have to do this. Sweetheart, it's okay. We're going to figure this out. Don't worry, my Angelhead."

I wanted nothing more than to comfort him. My poor baby Angelhead.

Maybe therapy isn't the answer. I mean fuck, *how the fuck was all of this scheduling stuff helping us? It wasn't. Fuck Patti. She was making things worse.* I fumed to myself. I'd never seen John like this before.

But I calmed myself down. I knew blaming Neutral P. wasn't the answer. In the past, therapy had not helped me in the way I thought it would or at the rate I thought it should. But it had, I had to admit, been of help in ways I never would have thought, at times I never would have suspected.

thirteen

the eternally suffering collapsible beauty boy

It was the Eternally Suffering Collapsible Beauty Boy who told me I should go into therapy in the first place. Of course I thought his suggestion was ridiculous. I'd always thought it was just for people like him—Woody Allen types with chronic headaches, irritable bowels, insomnia, depression, and divorced parents.

I'd never met anyone like the ESCBB. His name was Evan and his desperation to be cool certainly rivaled mine. He was more of a geek in high school than I was, so I think it's fair to say his desire for coolness was greater than mine, and, to his credit, he was more successful at it and remarkably aware of what fueled his need. The only thing I had up on him was living in New York—and for such an avid Woody Allen fan, that was hard to beat. But Evan made do with creating a James Dean–inspired, old-school Hollywood life that intrigued me as much as it obsessed him. He had an old Harley, a vintage Ford Falcon that never worked, a classic 1920s apartment with a strained view of the Hollywood sign, an ever-growing CD collection that showed off his highly cultivated eclectic musical tastes (even though he almost exclusively played Leonard Cohen and Elvis Costello), acclaim for a great performance in a cult film, a sitcom deal with CBS, a chiseled torso, shoulders covered in tattoos, a debilitating depression, a

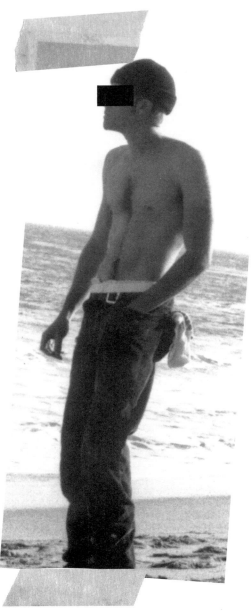

I would never be able to compete with Eternally Suffering Collapsible Beauty Boy's suffering. Never.

black leather jacket, a sharp mind, a rare sense of humor, a broken heart (that I thought I could repair), and a tall, thin body that became so amazingly small when he sat on the floor with his knees clutched to his chest that I was inspired to insert "collapsible" into my nickname for him.

And he seemed almost as, if not just as, intrigued by my life as a not-so-struggling artist in New York. Our first night together, he lay down on his chic grungy 1940s sofa and listened and listened and listened and listened as I carried on about my latest art project that I'd prosaically entitled *Boxes*. Impressed by his sense of style and successful life, I did my best to impress right back.

What I'd done this time was create an elaborate system of labeled boxes that housed all kinds of mail just so I'd have an excuse to design an "owner's manual" where, in order to illustrate how the project worked, I could quote from correspondence that had had a profound effect on my life. Such as the note from my mom that detailed my summer's expenses and how much I would owe her in theory. Or the love letter from Dylan in which he pondered how "different" the sexual aspect of our relationship was. Or the postcard from Auggie telling me he loved me only after we'd broken up. Or an overdraw notice from my bank, evidence of my irresponsibility with money. (Later, I'd include a disappointingly brief, matter-of-fact note from Evan that accompanied the clothes he was returning to me by mail after he broke up with me.)

Soon I was spending night after night at Evan's, which I preferred to driving home to my parents in the Valley after a night out with him in Hollywood. And then one day, without an invitation, I brought over most of my clothes, unofficially moving in. Knowing I'd be returning to New York at the end of the summer took the pressure off the appearance of our relationship progressing too quickly.

The next two months of our time together were punctuated with tantrums, crying, and desperation because I wasn't getting the love I wanted from Evan, compounded by so many years of not getting the love I so desperately wanted/couldn't handle. However, I wasn't playing with an amateur. Evan's antics were a sure match for my own. His painful headaches and gastrointestinal bouts on the toilet always trumped my need for attention. I wanted him to love me as much as he professed to love the girl who had broken his clearly still-broken heart. Why (oh why) would he want Sara when he could have me? Hadn't he said that they had long since stopped having sex? And wasn't I there, ready to be the sex kitten I thought he wanted, even though he didn't really show any signs of wanting it? Why did he ignore me—me, his new girlfriend—at parties? Why didn't he want to make out very often? Why did he still want to stay with me if he didn't want to hang out with me at parties or kiss? It never occurred to me to ask any of the questions I had directly. All I could do to communicate was cry.

"What's wrong, Jennifer? You can tell me. Just tell me," he'd plead.

But I couldn't manage to actually articulate any of the pain I felt.

"You should see a therapist," he'd say.

I *don't need a therapist*, I thought. I *just need you to love me.*

I was hoping Evan would be unduly impressed with me and my art project that I claimed was about "correspondence" but was really about love.

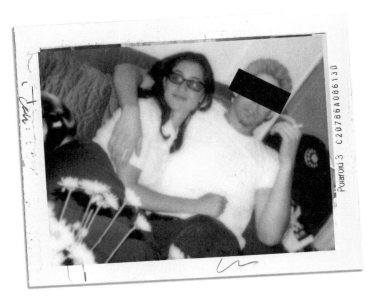

Me and the ESCBB at the height of our "honeymoon period," which lasted about twelve hours—if that.

As our relationship continued to disintegrate, his ex-girlfriend Sara who had broken his not-yet-healed heart came back into our lives just in time to help my misery reach its climax. Sara had been hired as a guest star on that week's episode of the sitcom Evan was on and he was furious about it. So furious that he had to spend every minute consumed with her while I spent every minute consumed with him being consumed with her. He had to talk to Sara on the phone for hours about how could she do this to him? My patience long since tried, I was hysterical at being so cast aside, at being so totally unable to compete. And he couldn't take my hysterics anymore. I was too much. It was over.

Rejected and beyond down-and-out, I had to go stay with my parents until my plane ticket said I could go back to New York, three days of non-stop crying later. I slept in my sunglasses and was mortified that my parents had to see me in such pathetic condition. When I called Evan in a desperate attempt to undo the breakup, he could only (once again and more pronouncedly) urge me to do what he'd been urging me to do for nearly the entire summer: go to therapy.

Back in New York, I was miserable. I hated my job as an assistant to this very unstable, verbally abusive woman/terribly tacky artist who was so prone to flying off the handle when things weren't done the way she wanted, the second she wanted, that even the postal workers closed their windows when they saw she was next in line. And the pain of knowing that

Evan would rather not have me in his life than have me in his life continued to excruciate. Months of discomfort later, I finally mustered the nerve to ask my friend to ask her boyfriend for a therapist recommendation, which is how I ended up on the Upper West Side talking to a woman with a head full of poodlelike hair.

But it didn't seem that this therapy stuff was going to be of much help. Poodlehead would just sit there and say very little as I told her how hard it was to see Evan in TV *Guide*, and how miserable I was working for the bitch who had five lawsuits pending at once. I had no idea how what we were doing was going to help me get over Evan—which was, I naively thought, the purpose of therapy.

As our biweekly sessions droned on, I decided to apply to graduate schools in art. I'd been in New York for four years and was starting to understand how hard it would be for me to break into the hip, cliquish, seemingly impenetrable art world that I convinced myself was the right place for me. Graduate school would allow me to leave New York with grace and purpose. It would buy me another few years to get my life together. And I hoped my work would finally get the critical feedback I craved.

While I applied to seven schools, I really wanted to go to UCLA. It was the Yale of art schools and was quickly building a reputation of turning out the latest hot young art stars. It was, I hoped, just the entrée I needed into the art world. And if pressed, I had to admit to myself that it would also bring me back to the city where the Eternally Suffering Collapsible Beauty Boy lived. Even though it was more than over, I still harbored fantasies of us getting back together.

Meanwhile, I dulled my Evan-doesn't-love-me pain by creating elaborate, hopefully compelling applications that took months to complete.

fourteen

lots of wondering

UCLA did send me the We're-pleased-to-inform-you letter I'd been hoping for. I immediately called my parents with the good news. Congratulations were offered and accepted. Underneath all of the well-wishing, however, I wondered what my parents really thought of me going to get a master's in "New Genres," of all things. Did they wonder what I was actually going to do with my degree? Did they wonder how much longer it meant they'd have to help support me? Did they regret encouraging my artistic pursuits all these years? Was graduate school just an excuse to not get a job job? Were they being bamboozled? Was I bamboozling?

And while I wondered what they wondered, I never asked. And if they wondered any of the things I was pretty sure they were wondering (but hoped they weren't), I never heard about it. Instead, I kept everything very "Isn't it great I got into such a prestigious program that only accepts two or three students a year in my discipline?" and they kept everything very "Yes, it's really a great accomplishment."

Our approach worked decently enough until it was time for me to buy a car. Even though I wanted an SUV, I knew that, as an art student with no job, I had no right to one. So I told my parents I would be looking for a used Volvo station wagon in the *Recycler*, hoping to find one for around five thousand dollars (which of course I'd need them to pay for). My parents didn't say one way or the other if they thought my price was what they were willing to spend.

My dad volunteered to help me with my search. Looking in the *Thomas Guide* for neighborhoods we'd never heard of in order to find a car that we'd have to drive to a mechanic to get checked out during a heat wave was not my dad's idea of car shopping. So we climbed into his Lexus and drove to a used-car lot where we found a SUV for ten thousand dollars. "That's not so bad," I was surprised to hear my dad say, considering it was double what I had guessed they'd feel comfortable spending. "Oh, but it has a hundred thousand miles! That's too many," he said.

Then, when we found another SUV with eighty thousand less miles on it for just four thousand dollars more, we called my mom to see if we should consider it. Without directly saying yes or no, she recommended we have it checked out by a mechanic. It turned out the low price tag was due to an accident the car had been in.

Just for the fun/education of it, my dad wanted to check out some new cars. After visiting a bunch of lots, we found one brand-new Rodeo for just $16,999. Rounding $999 down, my dad noted, "Just two more thousand dollars for a brand-new car with warranties!" Unfortunately, it didn't have a stereo, air bags, power anything, or even air-conditioning. Worn-out by the outrageous heat, the never-ending sales pitches from the desperate, sweating salesman, and a search with no parameters, we went home for a break.

We gave my mother the full report, and she was not remotely happy with our progress. Five thousand had become ten, then fourteen, then seventeen—and that was *without* tax and license. Our shopping was getting out of control! Panicked, but not without other resources, I did what I'd done so many times before: I called my grandparents.

"Hi, Grandmother."

"Well, hi, Jennifer. How is the car shopping? It must be hard in this heat."

"Well, we found this great, used SUV for fourteen thousand and it only had something like fifteen thousand miles on it. Unfortunately, we found out it had been in an accident."

"Well, I'm not surprised. You just don't know what you're getting with a used car. We don't buy used cars in this family."

"Well, we did look at new cars, too, but they were, as I'm sure you can imagine, considerably more."

"Let me talk to your grandfather and I'll call you back."

Minutes passed and then the phone rang.

"Oh, hi, Grandmother . . . I'm sure it would, Grandmother, thank you so much. I'll go talk it over with my parents."

"Hi, Mom, I just got off the phone with Grandmother and they offered to contribute five thousand dollars to my car. Will that help?"

"Well, oh my goodness, isn't that generous of them? What a surprise! Well, yes, that certainly does make a difference."

I went into the den to report the good news to my dad. We had started to discuss the possibility of purchasing the sixteen-thousand-dollar-plus Rodeo when my dad wondered why we would spend so much money on a car that didn't have air-conditioning or air bags? It seemed like a lot of money for a car that couldn't properly protect me from the sun or an accident. My dad said we should go back to the lot and see what the safer, more comfortable Rodeos went for.

Nineteen thousand was the answer. Nineteen *plus* tax and license. As we walked off the lot, my dad asked me which color I'd like to have if I could have any color. "Silver," I told him.

"Twenty thousand dollars! Now this really is getting out of control!" my mother said as if the president was considering starting a war. "This is just getting beyond me. I have in no way prepared our finances for an expenditure of this kind. It would take me a long time to put away money for this type of purchase."

Totally worn-out and dejected, my dad and I went and sat in the den.

"Dad, this isn't worth it. Why don't we just go back to considering a used Volvo wagon?" I offered, trying to make everything right.

Frustrated that he'd wasted a week of his life that could have been spent playing tennis in Malibu just to have his daughter wind up with a car he wouldn't want to get into, my dad had reached his limit. "Am I not a successful art dealer? What have I worked so hard my whole life for? To not buy my daughter a car with air bags for an extra few thousand dollars? All of this over a couple grand? This is ridiculous!" With my dad's meltdown and her parents' contribution, my mom agreed to the purchase. For the fifth time in two days, my dad and I drove over to the dealership and just bought me the goddamned car.

I felt guilty and elated. Was I a spoiled brat? Was this drama my fault because I didn't have a real job and was going to get a bullshit art degree? Was this the price I had to pay for not having my life together yet, when I so clearly should have had it together by then? I suspected that my mother thought so, even though I didn't accuse her of thinking of it and she didn't accuse me of being a leech.

(It never occurred to me to wonder why my parents hadn't sat down together to discuss what they both thought was the maximum amount they felt comfortable spending on a car for me, if indeed they felt comfortable doing it in the first place. It didn't dawn on me that they should have had a united front, seeing that it was their money and their daughter.)

The next day I took the car over to my grandparents to thank them in person. I took them for a spin, and when they got out, I told Grandmother to push down the lock and hold the handle up because I didn't have power locks.

"No power locks?" she exclaimed, shocked some cars still came without them.

"Grandmother, that would've been an extra thousand dollars," I explained.

"You should have told me! You need power locks!" she said, not aware that I had never in my whole life of asking her for things actually asked for the things directly. It would sound like I was trying to get something from them, as if I was only coming to them for their money. I'd learned that the approved-of way to get what I wanted was to share my problems as if I was only looking for emotional support. Not surprisingly, when you rely upon a method of indirect communication, things inevitably fall through the cracks.

One week later I was plagued with buyer's remorse. I shouldn't have let it happen. I chastised myself for wanting it to. The route to getting it was not worth it.

There I was, back in L.A. with my fancy car and guilty feelings—eager to start school already. While I had to admit to myself that I did harbor hopes of getting back together with Evan, I hoped even more that I'd find some fellow art student so great that I'd finally move on without batting an eyelash.

fifteen

the studios

Art school was no different from other school/ work scenes, in that there were cliques and loners. Dependable people and flakes. Nerds and cool people. Ass kissers and could-give-a-shitters. Some did drugs, some didn't. Some dressed hip, some dressed hippie. Some went grunge, a few went clean and pretty. Some professors were famous, some were jealous. Some had tenure, some were desperate for it. Some students dated each other unabashedly, some hid their affairs. Some students worked for professors. Some students who worked for professors also fucked the professors they worked for. Sometimes those students got gallery shows. And some students just got fucked over. And it was all grist for the gossip mill.

Tom was a not-very-tall painter who wore dark Levi's with an untucked oxford, had a superfull head of loose, Italian curls, and sported too-big-for-his-face glasses. He was friendly with some of the people I was friendly with, and we all made plans to meet for a drink one night. But in the end it was only the two of us—just as I had secretly hoped—who made it to the hipster, dimly lit Los Feliz bar.

One vodka grapefruit in, we soon discovered he was heartbroken and I was heartbroken. We had a great time.

Jennifer Lehr

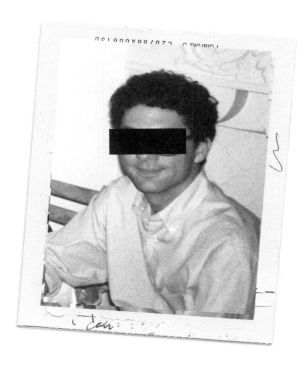

Tom was upset, and I was upset. We had a great time.

I listened to him tell me how upset he was over Penny, and about how little she cared about him, and I said similar stuff about the Eternally Suffering Collapsible Beauty Boy. There we were telling each other how much we were unloved by those we loved—meanwhile, flirting. I was in rare first-real-conversation-in-a-bar-seduction form, and I enjoyed it so much. But wait, did he say Penny? The short, mousy, slightly pigeon-toed, keep-to-herself girl in the sculpture department? Her? He was so upset over her?

Hours later, I was conveniently way too drunk to drive home. Tom probably was, too, but he lived close by and was willing to risk it. "You can stay at my place . . ." he started to say. When we climbed into his big old truck, he finished his thought: ". . . *if you promise not to tell anyone.*" I promised as if his request wasn't odd and insulting. So he drove us back to his little house in Silverlake.

Tom gave me a big T-shirt as pajamas and offered me his bed. He'd be sleeping on the sofa in the living room, he explained. *What? The sofa? He's sleeping on the sofa—and I'm not supposed to mention this to anyone?* "Let's sleep in your bed together," I suggested, stating what I thought was the obvious. So he climbed in and just lay there on his back, staring at the ceiling. He actually thought that we—two drunk, single, mid-twentysomethings—could manage a platonic sleepover. Feeling rejected, I whispered my interest in a kiss. And then boom, he was at it—fast and hard. Soon there was a pillow under my back and a finger up my ass, which brought me to a much-louder-than-he-was-comfortable-with orgasm.

"Shhhh, be quiet," he whispered as I climaxed. "My roommate is sleeping in the next room." This guy was interesting.

The next morning he had to once again make clear that what happened—which he made sure wasn't actual him-inside-of-me S-E-X—was between him and me. *Why*, I wondered, *couldn't I be with someone who didn't mind/was happy for someone to know he likes me*? But I was undeterred. Undeterred and unhappy. Unhappy enough to once again follow the ESCBB's advice.

sixteen

drawing my face

Wendy was a surprisingly young therapist who was just embarking on her own practice. She dressed very poor man's Ralph Lauren, and was an attractive woman except during those not-so-occasional moments when her eyes popped unnaturally far out of their sockets. Then she wasn't so cute anymore. Unable to not study her "condition," I noticed that her eyes bulged out when she was either trying to show empathy, or was tired and was forcing herself to listen extra hard. Anyway, I liked her more than Poodlehead. With her, therapy was more of a conversation.

I went twice a week and reported on my pursuit of happiness with Tom, "I simply do not understand why Tom is still so interested in Penny when he can be with me. I mean, he slept over at my place earlier in the week and we had such a wonderful breakfast in the morning. He cut up the mangoes like a gourmet chef. I mean, he's always telling me how uncaring she was. How unsupportive of his work she was. How competitive she was. Well, I'm not like that at all! What's the problem with being my boyfriend? How hard could it possibly be? I mean, one minute we'll be sitting in his truck on a side street, talking and talking. And then the next I hear *his* voice coming from *her* studio." The Eye-Popper would listen and listen. And sometimes she'd ask me some questions that led me to seemingly unrelated stories. I'd find myself talking about my mom and dad or telling her about the ESCBB and Sara. And I'd leave feeling like I wasn't getting anywhere, wondering how therapy worked.

My awareness of how crazy-making Tom's behavior was didn't keep me from coming back to him for more. On the contrary, I had a drive to win him—once and for all. God forbid I actually be in school and not have a Bobbie or a Nick-the-Eye-Flutterer to distract me from my work. Fortunately for my sanity, I was seized by inspiration. I had an idea for a new project.

I designed an invitation that I sent to every student and faculty member in the MFA program, asking if they'd please participate in my new project by coming to my studio to draw my face and to let me draw theirs. I included an appointment card so they could let me know when it was convenient

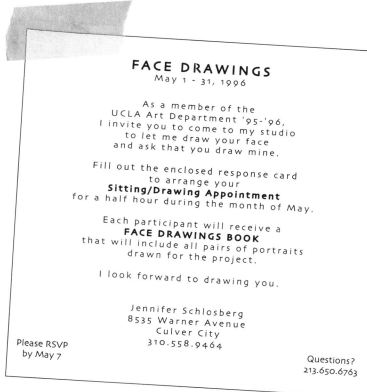

FACE DRAWINGS
May 1 - 31, 1996

As a member of the UCLA Art Department '95-'96, I invite you to come to my studio to let me draw your face and ask that you draw mine.

Fill out the enclosed response card to arrange your **Sitting/Drawing Appointment** for a half hour during the month of May.

Each participant will receive a **FACE DRAWINGS BOOK** that will include all pairs of portraits drawn for the project.

I look forward to drawing you.

Jennifer Schlosberg
8535 Warner Avenue
Culver City
310.558.9464

Please RSVP
by May 7

Questions?
213.650.6763

for them to come. I also explained that as a thank-you for their participation, each person would receive a book with all of the drawings. However, I added on the rsvp card, should you choose not to participate, please know that your page in the book will be blank—with your name on it. I was surprised that some saw this caveat as a threat—as if the worst thing in the world was to have your name on a blank piece of paper in my *Face Drawings* book.

I never would've dreamed that such a benign project would cause me and so many people at school such heartache.

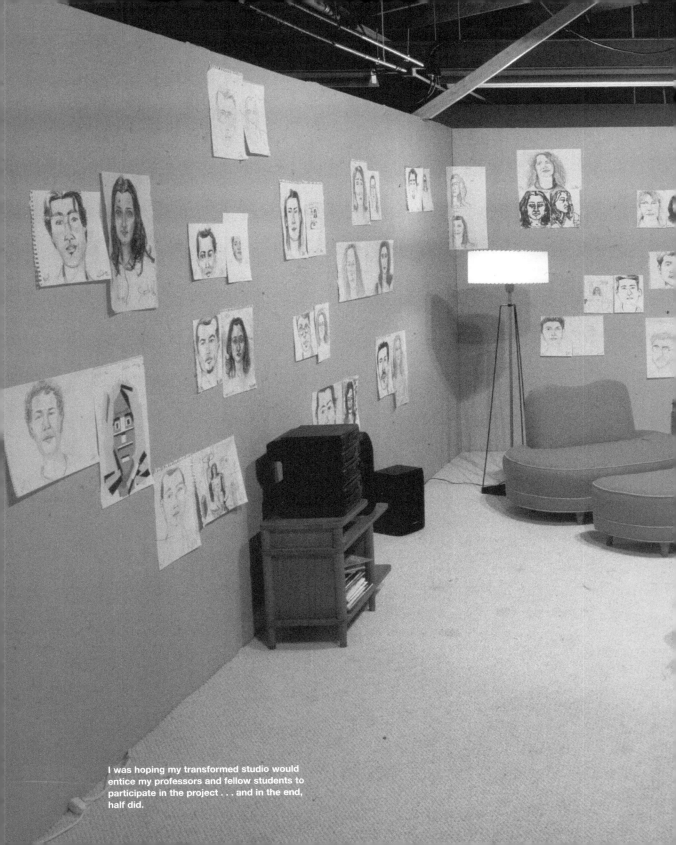

I was hoping my transformed studio would entice my professors and fellow students to participate in the project . . . and in the end, half did.

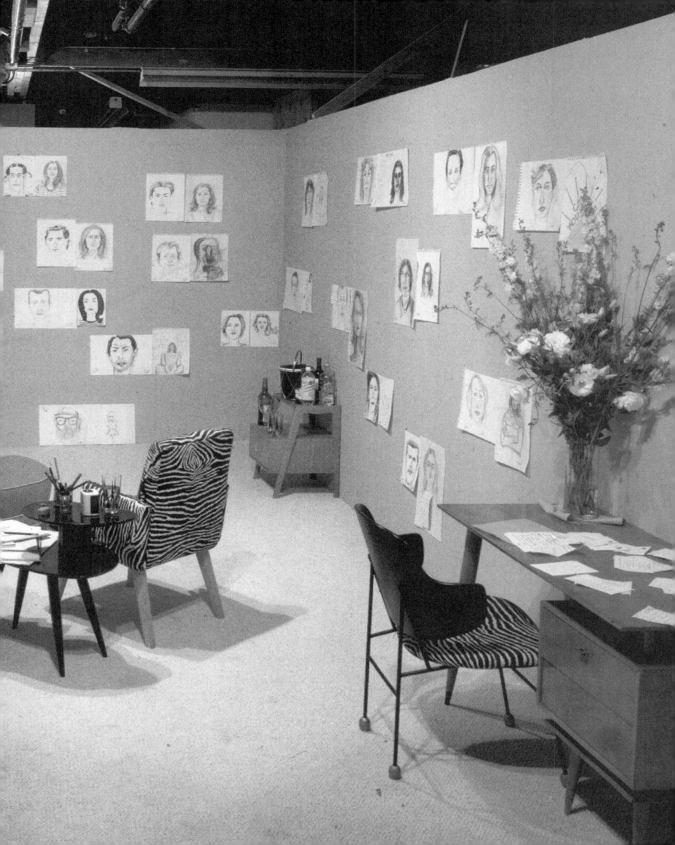

Actually, I saw my project as rather benign, if not outright friendly. We all had so many preconceived notions about one another based on what people wore, what type of work they made, which professors liked their work, whether or not they'd already received gallery interest, and with whom they hung out. Drawing each other's faces was an opportunity to get to know each other in a different context. With *Face Drawings*, I was setting out to illustrate that we are all more alike than we think. We all have two eyes, a nose, a mouth, and if we can strip away the other stuff, we might find we like one another more than we assumed.

Like many a party giver, I sent out my invites, nervous that no one would RSVP.

Soon the rumors were flying. I heard that some people were accusing me of using my project as a way to procure drawings from the famous faculty to later sell! Others thought I was trying to lure the famous faculty to participate just to raise the profile of my project so that I could masquerade their drawings as an endorsement of my work. *Face Drawings* as a career move. Others had me pinned as a total loser who was desperately trying to make friends via my art project. Some wondered if it was cool to participate, or cool not to. Should they acknowledge my invite when they saw me, or should they act like they never received it—as if I wasn't waiting to hear from them? Should I ask people if they were going to make an appointment, or should I not put them on the spot?

Meanwhile, I had transformed my studio from the standard grunge work space to a chic Shangri-la. While I was hoping an inviting setting would entice people to participate, I had to admit that it was also an excuse to decorate. I found myself loving to vintage-furniture-shop and my studio was a perfect blank slate to experiment on. Meanwhile, every day I couldn't wait for the mail to see who had sent in their appointment cards.

Soon the project was up and running and people were showing up for their drawing sessions. After we finished our drawings, my guest would hang them on the wall in my studio. People would stop by to see the drawings as well as to see who was and wasn't participating. I heard that on-the-fencers were anxious to see if any of the "big guns" had participated—to see if it was worth bothering.

Double-meanwhile, the drama between Tom and me had become excruciating. My drawing sessions were my only relief because they forced me to concentrate on someone and something other than the feelings of confusion, rejection, and pain that our poor excuse for a relationship was inflicting on me. One day I was so worn-out from it all that I even fell asleep while a fellow student was drawing me. I felt terribly rude—not even able to be awake for my own project. As the allotted month for my drawing project was coming to a close, and I had yet to receive Tom's response card, I asked him if he was planning on coming. I was hoping that at least my project could get him to sit in a chair and talk to me. Not now, he told me. Drawing my face, he seemed to imply, was simply making our relationship too public. Penny would then know he was sleeping with me is what he didn't quite manage to say, using absolutely no logic. I was enraged. How could he give me head—while I had my period, no less—yet not draw my face? Wasn't he Mr. Art-is-the-most-important-thing-in-the-world?

The rejection was driving me crazy. My tears were uncontrollable. I often found myself driving around the city alone in my car, crying and crying—the poster child for the Red Hot Chili Peppers' song that often played on the radio at the time, "Sometimes I feel like my only friend is the city I live in, the City of Angels . . ." Many nights I cried myself to sleep—but not with quiet whimpers. No, I howled. One of my neighbors even complained to another neighbor, without a trace of sympathy, that my crying had kept her up. Sticking up for me, my neighbor had responded with, "Maybe her grandma died." But nothing so terrible had happened, so I couldn't understand why I was crying as heavily and as long as I was. It's not like Tom and I had been dating for years and my life was falling apart without him. Nonetheless, I found my-

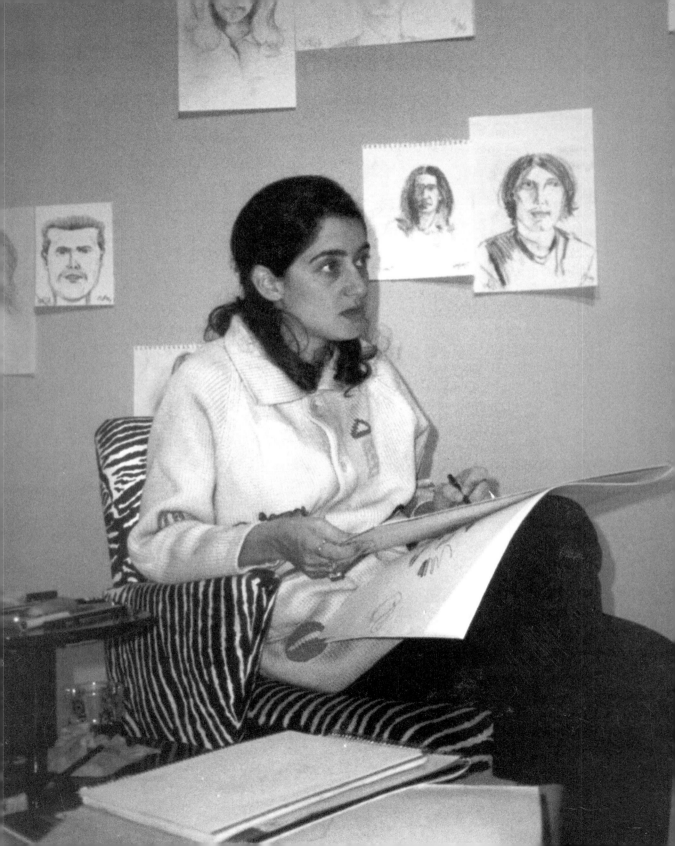

self waking up in the middle of the night, screaming, tears rushing down my face, with only my pillow to comfort me. Like a good patient, I reported my crying to the Eye-Popper.

"Have you experienced this type of crying before?" she asked.

"Well, yeah, actually, when I lived in New York, a couple of times I woke myself up in the middle of the night crying, not aware that I'd had a bad dream."

"Did you cry a lot as a child?"

"Well, yeah. Apparently from a very early age, I was a tantrum thrower. I'd just go all out, kicking and screaming and crying as hard as I could."

"And how would your parents respond?"

"Um, well, I was sent to my room a lot. 'Crying is just fine,' they'd tell me, 'as long as you do it in your own room.' "

"It seems they had a hard time sitting with your feelings."

"What do you mean?"

"Well, when you were upset, when you were very upset, your parents sent you to be by yourself. They didn't seem to stay with you long enough to work through your feelings with you, or to let you know that it was okay to feel upset, or angry, or misunderstood. The message your parents might have been giving you was that if you felt 'negative' or 'inappropriate' or 'disruptive' feelings, that you had to feel them alone."

"Oh. But you don't know my mom and dad. You couldn't ask for more loving, devoted parents than mine. Growing up, I always felt like I was the light of their life."

"Jennifer, I'm not saying they were bad parents or that they didn't love you. It is very clear that they have always loved you very, very much. It's just that they might not have had the parenting skills to help you work through your feelings. That doesn't mean they were bad parents. It's just that feelings weren't their strength. And therefore, now as an adult, it is an area we have to work on here."

I wasn't so thrilled when I found in my mailbox Penny's appointment

I was hoping Tom would come draw my face, but as it turned out, he could only give me head.

card with an X in the "Yes, I'd like to draw your face and have you draw mine" box. There was a note on the back—one I dreaded reading. She gave me two times for the appointment, whichever one worked best for me, please let her know. But before Penny and I could have our appointment, she decided she wanted Tom back. She now finally felt she was ready to get married. Well, this was more than I could take. That bitch. She couldn't have cared less until I started to care.

Desperation. Anger. Shock. No light at the end of the tunnel. The Eye-Popper's eyes were constantly popping with empathy as I related my story of woe. She listened carefully and asked me some questions that led to more of the same old Tom & Penny stories, Dad & Mom stories, Evan & Sara stories, and then I started to add some stories I haven't bothered to mention here because they were so goddamned repetitive. Stories starring people with names like Jeremy & Corey, Geoff & Amy, Doug & Carrie. And I'd drive home in tears, uncontrollably sobbing as I made my way through traffic.

In the end, thirty-nine people showed up to draw—exactly half of the seventy-eight invited. Now I was trying to keep my mind off of Tom, who had once and for all told me it was over (while dry-humping me in a very erotic breakup session) by designing my fancy gatefold book full of the drawings and blank pages. But in the end I was frustrated by how uncommunicative my *Face Drawings* book was. I had felt so many feelings and thought so many thoughts about who did and didn't come and what the drawing sessions were like, and all I had to show for it was a well-designed book of quickly rendered drawings. Encouraged by one of my professors, I decided to write a book about the experience—something I'd never even thought about thinking about. I turned on my computer and sat down to write a chapter on each person, exploring why I thought they did or didn't draw my face.

My suspicions, paranoia, fear, longing, and sadness poured onto the page. Uncensored, I let myself write every single thing I thought.

seventeen

oh

Soon the word got out I was writing a book about everyone at school, and so my project expanded. For the next nine months, I chronicled everyone's response to my response to their response to my invitation to draw my face. It was a rough, thrilling time. Some people were absolutely outraged by what they called my gossip rag despite the fact they hadn't read a word I'd written. It was immoral to write about people. Unethical. Hurtful. A couple of professors stopped talking to me. One even asked me to drop his class on my voice mail.

Finally, for the first time, I'd mustered the courage to explicitly express myself, and where did it land me? More alone than ever. *What was I supposed to do? Make art that didn't express myself?* I wondered. Some students ignored me in protest. I was called a bunch of names behind my back that didn't take long to find their way to me. What surprised me most was that this deluge of fear/anger/outrage over my art project was coming from some of the most—if not *the* most—hard-core, progressive, avant-garde artists in the country. When my work was weak, I didn't get much feedback. When it was strong, I was vilified. But I was undeterred. Five hundred single-spaced pages and lots of drama later the newly christened 78 *Drawings of My Face* was finished, or at least abandoned.

I had a lot of questions for the Eye-Popper. Why had I created a project that was making people hate me? Was it/I really unethical/immoral? Was there a difference between the two? Was I really bad/mean/uncaring/vengeful person? What was art supposed to do, not express feelings? What wasn't I allowed to say?

"Jennifer, do you remember how your parents responded when you shared your most 'inappropriate' yet honest feelings? When you threw tantrums? When you were too much?" the Eye-Popper asked, her eyes in rare popping form.

"Yeah . . . they put me in my room."

"Well, it seems that your book is similar. When you are finally expressing your truest feelings, ones that aren't particularly 'nice,' what happens?"

"People don't want to talk to me."

"That's right. I think your project is replicating this very primal experience you had as a child . . . this need to be heard, this need to be understood—whatever the cost."

Mmm . . . I was impressed with the Eye-Popper's take on my work. It certainly was more than I was getting from most of my highfalutin professors.

And more than anything, what I wanted to know was why (the fuck) did Tom want Penny over me, when it seemed that I was all of the things he wanted from her? Not only did I not see the contest, I couldn't understand why I wasn't the hands-down winner.

As usual, the Eye-Popper asked me a bunch of questions that I answered with extended stories. This droned on and on for months and months until one day I went, "Oh, wait." The chain hanging in the closet of my skull had been yanked. Somehow, by the art and science of psychotherapy, the Eye-Popper got me to realize on my own that (A) I was attracted to men who—while they truly liked and connected with me in a very special way—were attached to someone else, and (B) this particular "triangular relationship" (as the Eye-Popper later called it) I had with guys who were already attached to girls was shockingly similar to the relationship I had with my dad and mom. My dad and I related in so many ways that he didn't/couldn't with my mother. We were both aesthetic, we loved to shop, we had a similar sense of humor, we liked to take risks, and we both became frustrated with my mom/his wife not understanding us, particularly as fast as we understood each other. And so sometimes, when my mom didn't like a business risk my dad wanted to take, or the way he handled a situation, I'd explain to her why she was so small-minded, and then he'd chime in, becoming even more frustrated with her, and then my indignation would outdo his frustration. We'd feed each other's Mom's-way-of-seeing-the-world-is-wrong fire until I'd take it too far. Then my father would get mad at me for being rude and attacking his beloved, well-intentioned wife. How dare I talk to her/treat her like that! He'd defend his wife and turn against me. Just like Tom and Penny. Just like the ESCBB and Sara.

Why would he (Tom/Evan/my dad) *be with her* (Penny/Sara/my mom), my subconscious was apparently asking me, *when we* (Tom/Evan/my dad, and me) *got on so much better*? Penny/Sara/my mom would always be their number ones—not me. And there was simply and finally nothing I was able to do about it—no matter how attractive or smart or fun or sympathetic or manipulative I was. My dad was my dad, not my boyfriend. My mom was his wife, not some girlfriend. And so I'd automatically seek out a guy who absolutely would not, no matter how great it felt to be with me for a period of time, choose me over her. I was attracted to Tom/Evan precisely because he liked me very much but ultimately loved Penny/Sara more! I was doomed to perpetually be in a state of trying to win someone I'd never be able to have. On the other hand, apparently Derek, Dylan, Miknos, and Auggie were *too* unattached for me to want to be with them.

Well fuck, I'd never even thought to think about relationships like that before. Ever. I couldn't believe this was the way the human mind worked—let alone therapy. I was shocked and in awe. Why did the mind work this way? I wanted to know.

The Eye-Popper—surely proud of herself for successfully guiding me to this explosive breakthrough—tried to explain things to me in layman terms as best she could. She told me that the way we relate to our parents creates its own pattern. Early on in our lives, this pattern gets drawn onto our psyche. We respond to our parents in the same way, over and over and over and over and over and over and over and over again, and as we do, the pattern is drawn—like any path walked over and over again—creating tracks that get deeper and deeper. So if I could think about these tracks as imprinted on my brain, the Eye-Popper continued, it's only natural for me to continue to follow those tracks. It's always easier to walk on a previously created path than to try to hack out a new one. Sticking to the path feels safer and more familiar.

Wow. I was stunned. So this is how therapy works? I tell story after story after story, and my therapist sees a pattern and then (months and months or years and years later) gets me to see the pattern myself? Brilliant. How did I not know that? I drove home with so many thoughts, with so many synapses firing, that it felt like an electrical storm was lighting up my apparently previously unused brain. I started to look back on my life with an entirely new and informed perspective. All of my confusing-to-me-at-the-time stories quickly started to make sense.

I was reeling. I couldn't believe how deep my tracks were. What a waste of time my life had been not knowing about them.

Not too long after my revelation, the Eye-Popper told me she had something important to tell me.

"Jennifer, I wanted to take these last fifteen minutes of our session today to talk to you. Now, I want you to know that I know the timing isn't ideal, in terms of our work together, but I will soon be leaving my practice in Los Angeles."

"Why?" I barked as I crossed my arms.

"Well, I'm getting married."

"Congratulations," I forced myself to say.

"Thank you. Thank you very much. My fiancé lives across the country, so I'll be moving. However, this won't be for a month or so. I wanted to tell you now because I know you are struggling with issues surrounding people leaving you, particularly when you reveal your true self to them, so I thought we could use this as an opportunity to work through or make some progress with that issue."

"What? You want me to pay you to talk about you leaving me?" I was incensed. I was so angry during those last sessions I didn't open up enough to work through shit. She left me furious at her and at my parents and most definitely not the most popular girl at school. Now what was I supposed to do? I was boyfriendless, therapistless, and still waking up in the middle of the night wondering if I had, in fact, wronged my classmates.

eighteen

now what?

I didn't trust myself. Who was I supposed to date? Someone I didn't connect with, whom I wasn't attracted to, who wasn't fun to flirt with?

The Eye-Popper had left me with a bunch of therapist recommendations who, she had assured me, were in the same price range. And I was eager to find one (though resentful that I had to) because I wanted to know what I was supposed to do next. I met with three therapists—all of whom were at least fifty dollars more a session—whom I didn't like anyway. Worn-out from the interviews, and still angry at the Eye-Popper for abandoning me, I decided to take a little break from looking for a therapist. I promised myself, however, that in the meantime I'd be vigilant. No dating men still in love with someone else. Period. How hard could that be?

I'd try out my new resolve up at the pool of the hotel Chateau Marmont, just a few blocks from my house, where I liked to sneak in for a summer swim. My fantasy was that poolside, I'd meet some handsome, artistic man who was definitely single. Instead I found myself sitting on a lounge chair, having a friendly conversation with an extremely funny-looking Englishman with a crooked, long nose. Soon his lanky, Mohawked, gold-front-toothed friend joined him for a swim. Introductions were made and then I dove in after them.

Out of nowhere, I felt a distinctly palpable gravitational pull in the water. I had little choice but to swim as close to Mohawk Randy as possible without actually touching him. I pushed off the deep end and rocketed to the shallow end, which moved a mass of water that added some pressure around his ankle. I was flirting. Introductions and a minute in the pool was all it seemed to take. The crooked-nose guy, not realizing it wasn't he whom I fancied, wondered if I'd like to join them for cocktails in the garden later that evening.

Sitting on the rattan furniture, sipping my vodka grapefruit, my insides jumped when I saw Randy slink down the steps wearing his loose linen beige summer suit over an original tattered Sex Pistols T-shirt with Tevas. I'd never seen such a vision of beauty and style before.

The next morning—after our clumsy, unclimactic-for-me drunken screw at his hotel—was when I found out he had a gorgeous little three-year-old

While on the surface Randy wasn't the type of guy I usually went for, he actually was. It seems my big prerequisite for attraction was that the guy have a girlfriend.

daughter whose mother he'd been living with for the past twelve years. He admitted they both had a drug problem—though he didn't see it so much as a problem. He was a stylist for a big British rock band, and in his line of work, he explained, one had to take speed to keep up. Instead of berating myself for sending myself back to square one, I just told myself, *This was only a fling. He's not boyfriend material, so it doesn't count.* He lived in London. *Enjoy him while you can.* I

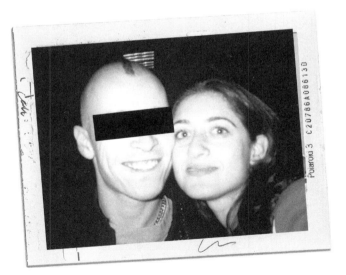

convinced myself it was OK because it felt so good to finally have some-one's arms around my shoulders talking to me sweetly.

A couple of nights later he said we'd go out after his dinner with business associates. So I waited by the phone as eleven, twelve, one, and two came and went. I was desperate for him and infuriated. The phone finally rang at some time after three. He was sloshed and so sorry, could he come over? "No," I forced myself to say. "I'll see you tomorrow." I had figured he hadn't called because his colleagues knew his girlfriend and he didn't want *me* to get back to *her*. While he was apologetic, I had had it with being the girl that had to be hidden from sight. I promised myself to be more vigilant. No more being with men who have women who are more important to them than I will ever hope to be.

Well, it wasn't as easy as one might think to determine if there was a girlfriend, ex or otherwise, lurking in the wings. Later that summer, I was invited out by an old friend to a birthday at a bar. Another pool table, another scotch, another cute guy, another successful flirtation. This time, however, I thought I got the information up front. **NO GIRLFRIEND.** No pining over a lost love. "Ready to date" was what I heard. The coast was clear. The evening ended with an exchange of e-mail addresses. I was hopeful.

The next day, he cleverly e-mailed me and I cleverly e-mailed back. Soon we were cleverly writing each other five times a day. But nowhere in his clever e-mails was an invitation out on a date. After a week or so of our clever bullshit, I finally asked if he wanted to get together. Turns out his more-important-than-me third party was his little girl, of whom he had sole custody. He was single, but taken. I should have known.

Coincidentally, around that time, I happened across a poem by Portia Nelson that made perfect sense to me. It likened the figuring-out-your-tracks-and-making-new-ones process to walking down a street with a hole in it:

AUTOBIOGRAPHY
in Five Short Chapters

I.

I walk down the street.

> *There is a deep hole in the sidewalk.*
> *I fall in.*
> *I am lost. . . . I am helpless.*
> *It isn't my fault.*

It takes forever to find a way out.

II.

I walk down the same street.

> *There is a deep hole in the sidewalk.*
> *I pretend I don't see it.*
> *I fall in, again.*

I can't believe I am in this same place.

> > *But, it isn't my fault.*

It still takes a long time to get out.

III.

I walk down the same street.

> *There is a deep hole in the sidewalk.*
> *I see it is there.*
> *I still fall in . . . it's a habit . . . but,*
> > *My eyes are open.*
> > *I know where I am.*
> *It is my fault.*
> *I get out immediately.*

IV.

I walk down the same street.

    There is a deep hole in the sidewalk.
    I walk around it.

V.

I walk down another street.

Well, me, I realized, I was still walking down the same street. I was seeing the hole but was still falling in. I was nowhere near walking down another street, let alone finding a new, safer neighborhood.

nineteen

(un)repentant

Afraid of walking down the same street with the same deep hole in it, I stayed home a lot. Gallery openings were emotionally draining, what with so many people ignoring me because of my book, and I was distinctly not being invited to parties thrown by my fellow students. So when my friend Daniella—whom I knew from New York—asked me to go with her to see her friend's band play at a club, I considered it despite the fact that I hate loud music and seas of people. A guy she was dating would be there and she didn't want to go by herself. *How bad could it be*? I wondered, encouraging myself to get out of the apartment.

While Daniella was off flirting with her game-playing, overwhelmed-by-his-own-beauty, Lenny-Kravitz-goes-to-Harvard type, I was left alone to be overwhelmed by the crowd, the music, and the colored lights flashing about. As I lamented my decision to deposit myself in the exact kind of place I knew I hated, I looked up at the balcony and noticed John Lehr sitting at a table with his friend Seth. John Lehr! I caught his eye, we waved furiously, and I quickly made my way upstairs.

John Lehr was the long-haired, alcoholic, chain-smoking, brilliant improviser/comedian/actor I'd met after I'd seen his I've-never-seen-anything-like-it-before show, back when I was dating the Eternally Suffering Collapsible Beauty Boy. I was happy for him when I'd heard through some mutual acquaintances that he'd recently gotten sober and quit smoking. Relieved to see a familiar face, I ran up the stairs to say hello and was greeted with a warm hug. After a round of "oh-my-Gods," "so-great-to-see-yous," and "how-are-yous," I was relieved to learn that he and Seth were leaving and were happy to give me a ride home.

When we pulled up in front of my building, I invited them in for a drink—eager for some company. Seth said he was sorry, he had to be up early for work, and John explained that his car was at Seth's. Quickly, I countered with an offer to drive John back to Seth's after our visit. John was sorry but it was just so late. However, he'd love to get together. He'd be sure to call me tomorrow. "Great," I said, totally disappointed that my evening was ending just when I thought it was going to get started.

As promised, John called the next day. How was I? Would I like to go out to dinner Saturday night? It was the closing night of his improv show and he thought we could have dinner, go to his show, and then go to a party afterward.

So the plans were set.

Even though I had gotten myself all dolled up, I honestly didn't think I was going out on a date date with John. Despite his immense talent and warm, welcoming disposition, John had dark circles under his eyes, wore oversized concert Ts, and still had long hair—long ever-so-slightly-thinning hair! He was an old acquaintance who I hoped would be a new friend. After the unofficial results came in that I was voted the least popular girl in grad school, I was hoping to make a friend in a whole other scene.

Saturday night came and John was late. Coming from Venice, he'd grossly miscalculated the traffic and didn't have a cell phone to call me with his ETA. So I anxiously (and increasingly angrily) paced my apartment, adjusting my hair and reapplying makeup, trying not to fume. After all, I was my grandparents' granddaughter, obsessed with being on time. But the second I saw John and his apologetic smile at my door, I forgave him. With no time for a proper meal, I recommended we grab a quick bite at Koo Koo Roo—a healthy fast-food place that I thought of as my personal chef. Dinner was quick. We tried to catch up, but were nervous we'd be late for his show, so we stuffed our faces, wiped our hands, and left. On the way to what I thought was the theater, dating came up and I lamented what a mess it was for me and how there was no one out there—not realizing John thought we were on a date.

"What am I?" he asked with a friendly laugh, nonetheless making his intentions clear.

"Gulp," I gulped. I wanted a friend, not someone whose feelings I'd hurt by not wanting to date him.

As it turns out, John wasn't driving us over to the theater, he was taking me home. Apparently, John thought we should take separate cars to the theater—though I didn't know why and didn't ask. Separate cars, however, were a point in the not-a-real-date column. Maybe John thought that after his show he'd have to clean up and break down the set, and thought I might not want to wait around, even though the set only consisted of three nursery-school-size chairs. All of our rushing landed us back at my place with some time to kill, so we took a walk around the block. I grabbed ahold of his elbow as we strolled, which John misinterpreted as a sign of interest. I was so not considering dating John that I felt comfortable enough to be affectionate. Arriving back at his car, I wished him luck and said I'd see him after his show.

I felt self-conscious walking up to the theater by myself. Didn't I look like a loser going out alone on a Saturday night—especially dolled up as I was in my knee-high black patent-leather boots and short navy swing skirt? I ended up being one of the last people inside the packed theater where only front-row seats were still available. That's when I saw John's movie-star friend who was also alone looking for a place to sit. *When you're famous*, I thought, *you don't look so much like a loser out alone on a Saturday night as much as you look cool, like you couldn't give a fuck*. I was excited when we wound up sitting next to each

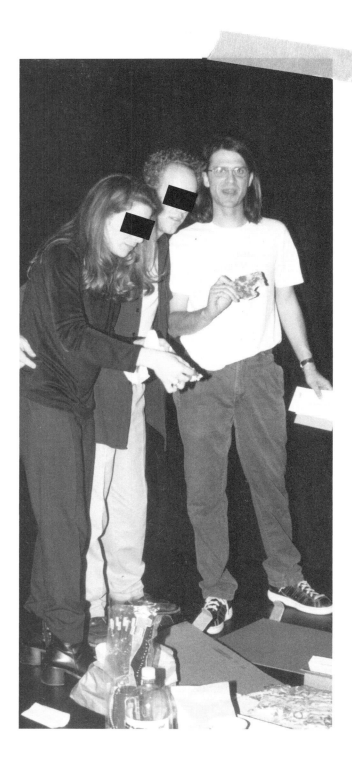

other, and I reintroduced myself, reminding him that we'd met at St. Nick's Bar when I was giving a reading from my book, 78 *Drawings of My Face*. Yes, he did remember, how was I? And then the lights went down and the show and the flirtation began.

It was pretty hard to detect at first. Was Movie Star's shoulder intentionally grazing mine when he leaned back laughing? Were our legs rubbing against each other when we were again jolted with laughter? The show was brilliant; John and his two partners were on fire. I couldn't imagine a better time—incredible entertainment and a sly flirtation with a handsome man. As the over-the-top, dark, funny, odd, crazy, smart show got more over-the-top, darker, funnier, odder, crazier, and smarter—Movie Star and I got braver and braver, rubbing our legs more, our shoulders harder. The back of our hands even touched when we were driven to some mid-performance applause. But we never went as far as a hand on a leg or anything. That would be

On my first official date with John, he performed with his improv group while I flirted with his movie star friend.

too far. Then it would be clear that we were actually doing what we were obviously doing but in a way that neither one could deny doing it. After the show, I shuffled out of the theater just in front of Movie Star as we small-talked briefly.

"Wasn't that a great show?" he said.

"Yeah, that was great," I said, wishing I could come up with something else to say.

There was a little wrap party in the lobby, so we hung out and struggled to have a conversation. I ended up carrying on about my landmark apartment building and the group of eccentric characters who lived there. He said I was like Jimmy Stewart in *Rear Window*. Coincidentally, I had just seen the movie the week before, so I got the reference and quickly responded with, "For all intents and purposes, I am Jimmy Stewart—minus the wheelchair, the murder, and a beautiful person falling in love with me." Didn't I look well versed in film classics? *For God's sake. Date me, I know what a cool movie* Rear Window *is.*

Movie Star said I was the Jimmy Stewart (in *Rear Window*) of my apartment building and I couldn't have agreed more. However, it didn't get me what I wanted— a date.

To get out of an awkward extended pause while trying to keep the flirtation alive, I jumped up on the bar behind me to get a better view of the party. That's when he turned toward me and I

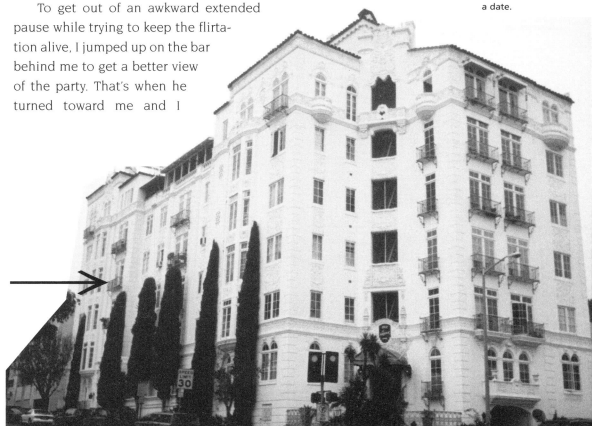

caught him looking up my skirt as I scooched my behind back. He knew I'd caught him peeking, and he said he was "unrepentant." *Nice vocab word*, I thought. I liked a sexy, handsome movie star looking up my skirt. Of course, if I hadn't seen him do things like fuck a stunning French actress playing a whore in an exciting bank-robbery-gone-wrong thriller, then I probably would have just thought he was a tacky, loser pervert with a terrible mustache whom I probably would have told to fuck off.

After his titillating comment, he turned around to face the party and leaned against the bar—between my legs. I liked how his fleece jacket felt against my inner thighs. As much as I loved it, it made me nervous. I didn't want any of John's friends to report us to John, who had yet to come out from backstage. Even though I was trying to convince myself that we hadn't been on a date date, I knew he liked me. How rude to have fun hanging out with him, go see him be brilliant in his show, and then spend the night flirting with his famous friend. Gross. But I liked the charge of being with Movie Star, not necessarily talking with him because conversation was strained at best. John was fun to hang out with, Movie Star was fun to flirt with.

And then, suddenly, Movie Star said good night. I thought for sure he was going to ask for my number, but he didn't. *Why was he flirting so much if he didn't want my number?* I wondered. Is that what movie stars did? Maybe he was planning to call John for it. At once I hoped he would; on the other hand, I hoped he wouldn't do that to his friend. I certainly wouldn't ask John for his. Ahhh, but I could ask my neighbor Peter, who knew Movie Star, too.

As it turns out, the night for John and me was over as well. There was a big party after and John said to go ahead, he'd meet me there, but he never showed up—at least, not by the time I left. Another point in the it-wasn't-a-real-date column.

Encouraged by this, the next day when I ran into Peter in the elevator, I tried to casually mention something about Movie Star. Peter told me he had a girlfriend. Didn't I know he dated So-and-So? Peter said they'd been together for something like eight years.

Of course! I thought. *What a fucking idiot I am. How many times do I need to be hit over the head with the same fucking stick? How was it so easy for me to forget that when I felt a strong, chemical, exciting, feeling-alive attraction that meant STOP! This guy is taken, despite his apparent interest in me—a get-me-nowhere combination.*

I marveled at the reality of the tracks I'd so deeply made with my mom and dad. I was shocked that I was still walking down the same goddamned street, not noticing the hole until I tripped and fell in. I thought I was being so vigilant. This time, however, I just climbed right out and kept going. I wondered about all the people who didn't go to therapy to find out what created their tracks. Were they just doomed to keep falling into an unhealthy relationship after unhealthy relationship? Are there other ways to find out what your tracks are without spending two years and twelve thousand dollars doing it?

I realized that quitting dating men I felt attracted to was going to be harder than quitting my pack-and-a-half-a-day-for-ten-years smoking habit. I didn't need two years of therapy to know that smoking could kill me, or at the very least radically ruin my life, yet it wasn't until two different people told me I was getting premature wrinkles that I finally stopped. Vanity made me quit. I wondered what was going to make me quit following that light-up-my-insides feeling that taken men ignited? Was I really ready to face a life of not having my insides light up ever again?

John called the next day to tell me what a great time he'd had, and that he was sorry he didn't go to the party but he was just so tired after the show.

"That's okay," I said, and meant it because I'd spent the entirety of the party talking to the Eternally Suffering Collapsible Beauty Boy and his not-so-new girlfriend. It was always fun to talk to him and a relief to not feel so much rage and rejection anymore—though I have to admit I couldn't help feeling that same old attraction. "You were incredible last night," I continued. "The show was really, really amazing. You guys couldn't be any better."

John soon steered the conversation around to its purpose. "Would you like to go out again? Maybe next weekend?" he asked.

There was no denying this was an official asking out for a real dee-ay-tee-ee date. I said sure. What was I going to say: *You're brilliant, funny, and fun, but you look like a troll*? Because he was going on a camping trip and because I was being flown by my sister to Oregon to decorate her new place in a four-day whirlwind, we couldn't get together for another three weeks. While I was looking forward to seeing him again, I could certainly wait the time our schedules dictated we had to wait.

twenty

a frog

I had been warned about the smell that permeated John's Venice beach house before I arrived. My friend Jason's friend Sam(antha) had recently gone out on a date with John, and while she thought he was very nice, funny, and talented, she wasn't so into John's struggling-actor-broke-substitute-teaching-in-South-Central scene and his package was made all the less appealing by the fact that his house smelled like cat piss. While Sam, I guess, was on the lookout for someone more successful, it had never dawned on me to have financial and career criteria for dating. The only criterion I had was that the guy not have a girlfriend or an ex he was still pining over. That was about all I could handle watching out for and clearly I hadn't handled it very well. Besides, I was looking for love, not marriage. Even though I was twenty-eight and finishing up my last year of graduate school, I wasn't even thinking about thinking about finding someone to marry.

John greeted me with a warm smile and a welcoming hug as his house greeted me with the stench of cat piss. John explained that unfortunately, no matter how hard you try, cat pee can never really come out of carpet. *Why have a cat, then*? I, someone raised by cat haters, wondered.

He gave me a tour of the beach house, introduced me

to his best friend/roommate Spunky and excused himself for a moment. Spunky was so friendly. So easy and fun to talk to. I liked the absence of too-coolness in these guys' lives and at the same time I missed it.

Soon we were off to Culver City because John wanted to stop by a wrap party for a children's TV show he did a guest appearance on—hoping, of course, they'd hire him again in the future. It was a weird scene. Little child actors dressed up like adults ran around the restaurant and played pool while their proud parents talked. The young star had an attitude, and so did a bunch of his friends—even I was intimidated by their confidence. John socialized with I'm not sure who for a bit, and when a little girl puked near my feet, I told John I'd be outside.

He thanked me for stopping by the party with him, and I told him it was my pleasure. We stopped for dinner at Café Brazil—a charming little order-at-the-counter restaurant with mismatched tables and chairs under an awning. Then ice cream. Then lattés. The entire evening was full of easy conversation, laughing, joking, sharing of artistic ambitions, life stories. No kissing, no hand-holding, no arm-arounds, no I-want-to-seduce-you feelings (on my part anyway), just talking and laughing and talking and laughing.

Our talking and laughing continued in the cat-piss-smelling living room. Then his other roommate, Richard, came home and joined in. The subject of dating soon came up—a safe topic now that a third party was present. After my self-deprecating I've-had-such-a-hard-time speech, John said that he couldn't believe it because I was such a catch. I lit up inside. He thought I was a catch, as opposed to someone whom he likes only after I've moved back to New York, or behind closed doors, or when his relationship is in trouble.

John then announced that he just couldn't stay up another minute, he was sorry, but he had to go to bed. He invited me to sleep over if I wanted, he knew it was late. I was welcome to sleep on the sofa or in the bed with him or he'd call me tomorrow. It was three in the morning and I wasn't sure what I should do or what I wanted to do, and if they were the same or different. To put off my decision making, I stayed in the piss room and talked to Richard for another half hour or so.

Close to four in the morning, it was clear I wasn't going to drive all the way back to West Hollywood, so I excused myself and went up to John's blank room. Aside from the futon and Lava lamp, the room was empty, save for an old valise that housed his boxers and socks. He was thirty-one living like he was eighteen.

I took off my skirt and climbed in bed with him. *Nothing would happen, right?* I tried to convince myself as if I weren't twenty-eight, as if I'd never done this before. I lay with my back to him. He scooted toward me for a spoon and we fell asleep.

In the morning he reassumed the spooning position as I shuddered to think of what was going to happen next. *Surely he won't try to kiss me without brushing his teeth*, I reassured myself. A first kiss with morning breath wasn't anyone's idea of romantic. But romantic or not, it's what he wanted. He gently turned me toward him and lifted me up on top of him and kissed me. And I kissed back. But I was so busy berating my stupid, unqualified-to-handle-myself self for once again landing me where I didn't want to be, doing something I didn't want to be doing, that I didn't notice if he had bad breath or not. I noticed nothing of the kiss. My mind raced only with my thoughts of what I'd gotten myself into and how I'd get myself out of it.

"Hey, let's get some coffee," I suggested.

Minutes later, I was awestruck by the outfit John found suitable to leave the house in: Birkenstocks; a soft, too small, army-green baseball cap that poofed out his long hair; yet another oversized T-shirt that made his small chest look the size of a ten-year-old's; and pants, sloppily cut off around the knee. He didn't have the sense of style to work the look in any other way than ridiculous goofball. *How*, I wondered, *did he expect me to find him attractive?* As we walked to coffee with Spunky and Richard, I was uncomfortable in my role of girl-who-slept-over-after-the-first-date even though they all probably considered it our second. I felt bad because I liked John Lehr so much, and

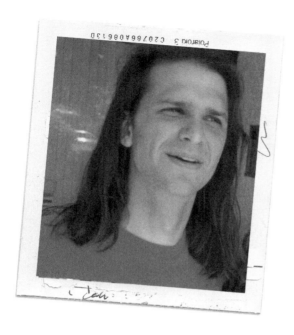

In an attempt to break things off, I told John the story of Miknos, by way of explaining how I had a habit of getting together with men I did not find remotely attractive because I felt guilty that I didn't find them attractive. Can you imagine anything more rude or hurtful?

now we wouldn't be able to be friends because he had a crush on me and I wasn't interested in dating him.

As if I had no control over myself, I went out on another date with John and wound up crying during the sex. Why was I crying? he wanted to know, and was frustrated because I couldn't be articulate. Sleep came, breakfast was a mood lifter, and off I went, once again, wondering how the hell I'd rectify this mess I'd gotten myself deeper into.

After thinking about it and thinking about it and thinking about it, I decided I owed it to John to be honest with him. I had to nip this in the bud. I had to do it right now before I lost my nerve. Without calling, I turned my car around and drove to Venice.

He was so happy to see me. What a great surprise. My impromptu visit probably said to him that I just couldn't wait to be with him again. We walked over to the beach as my nerve started to seep out of me. We walked back to the canals and I was still stalling. *Okay, you coward*, I said to myself, *put this poor guy out of his misery*.

I told John that I felt bad about how I had let myself rush into having sex the other day. Then, for some reason, instead of just saying, I *don't think this will work out*, I told him the expanded version of the truth. I told him I had a history of sleeping with men I wasn't attracted to because . . . well, instead of just telling him why, I told him the humiliating story of Miknos, by way of example. As I dug my hole deeper and deeper, basically comparing John's homely looks to Miknos's obesity, I couldn't take the pain I was surely inflicting on him another minute, so I used my lips as one would morphine. And if John was hurt by the hurtful things I was saying, he wasn't too hurt to kiss me back. If neighbors were walking by, they'd think we were two lovers stealing a passionate kiss under the beautiful moon.

I had good intentions but was having such a hard time becoming a better person. *Okay,* I said to myself once I was home, *absolutely no more dating men with girlfriends and no more sleeping with men you don't find attractive because you feel sorry for them. Before it was okay, you didn't know what you were doing, but now you do. So just don't do it!*

I confided in my friend Daniella who couldn't believe what I was saying.

"John Lehr is so cute! He's funny, supertalented, smart, warm, sweet, and he's definitely cute! He's sexy! How can you *not* find him attractive? You're crazy. You *must* give him another chance. At least one more date," she implored.

How can she think he's cute and sexy? I wondered. *Isn't he so obviously not cute and not sexy?* But then I thought, *Well, Mohawked gold-toothed Randy wasn't so objectively gorgeous, yet I thought he was so to die for. And even though Tom was pretty funny-looking, I adored his side smile. And there was a reason Evan usually played nerds and the best friend, never the lead. But God, I loved Evan's long fingers, his bunioned feet, and his long, skinny legs that held up his disproportionately pumped-up torso.*

I deduced that I found certainly-not-the-most-gorgeous men attractive because of my tracks, not their looks! I couldn't believe tracks had such transforming power. It was like light on color. Color wasn't intrinsic, it changed with light. Likewise, looks weren't intrinsic, they changed with tracks. And so maybe my unhealthy tracks made John's cute, sexy looks appear troll-like. Without the Eye-Popper around to verify my theory, I told myself I had to give this John Lehr a chance. So I forced myself to go out with him again. I was going to date him precisely because I was not attracted to him.

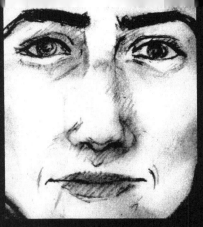
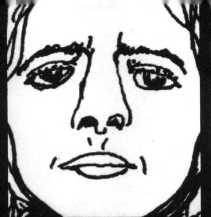
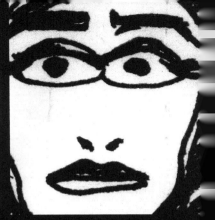
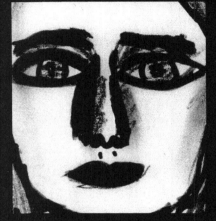

78

DRAWINGS
OF MY FACE

by
JENNIFER SCHLOSBERG

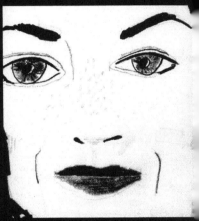
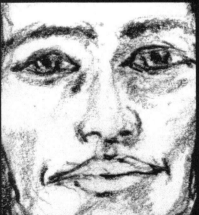
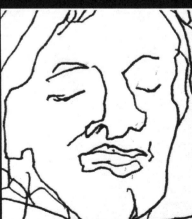
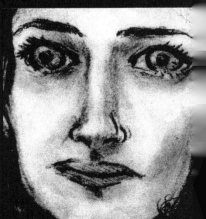

twenty-one

before we didn't do it

Soon after I finally shut my fear-filled, doubting self up and let myself date John without bringing up every ten minutes how I didn't think it would work out—it was his thirty-second birthday. My gift was a copy of 78 *Drawings of My Face*. I wanted him to see what he was getting himself into—to see the person I really was, uncut and uncensored.

A voracious reader who usually had four books going at any given time, John tore through 78 *Drawings of My Face*. He was the first person to read every single word. Each day he'd call and tell me which chapter he had just finished and which parts he liked best. He loved it. Loved it. He loved learning about the L.A. art scene that was so foreign to him, he loved my writing, and he loved my honesty. He loved learning about me! John wasn't afraid of all of my crazy thoughts and feelings. I loved it that he loved it so much.

We quickly became the typical I-must-talk-to-you-every-night-and-drive-over-to-your-house-at-10-P.M.-because-I-absolutely-cannot-go-to-sleep-if-I'm-not-in-the-same-bed-as-you couple falling in love. We had to be either on the phone with each other, on the way over to see each other (counting the minutes until we were together), or actually together. To my total shock, my frog

I gave John a copy of *78 Drawings of My Face* for his birthday so that he could see what he was really getting himself into with me.

had turned into a prince—a poorly dressed, not-exactly-handsome-but-definitely-getting-cuter-every-day prince.

Our sleepovers were difficult at first—but not because of sex.

John managed to make his way as a truly struggling actor in Hollywood by substitute teaching in the trenches of South Central high schools and by spending virtually no money on anything other than the bare essentials. Every morning at some ridiculous, predawn hour, he'd wake up to receive a phone call from the L.A. Unified School District assigning him to a school and room number for that day. He'd then shower, dress, grab his sack lunch, jump into his down-and-out Granada, and drive to the worst neighborhoods Los Angeles had to offer. That was his routine when he slept at his place. When he slept at mine, his schedule changed. To my shock, he'd set the alarm for 4:15 A.M. so he could drive back to Venice in time to get his daily call. I thought driving all the way across a city to answer the phone at the end of the twentieth century was absolutely absurd. I couldn't help but make a suggestion.

"What about call forwarding?" I asked.

"My roommates would then miss their calls. We only have one line. It wouldn't be fair," he replied.

"What about a cell phone?" I countered.

"Too expensive!" he rallied.

"What about leaving an outgoing message telling the assignment lady where she can reach you?" I said, keeping the volley alive.

"I don't want to inconvenience her. I don't want to give her a reason to skip over my name because locating me is too much of a pain in the ass. My life depends on that call," he slammed back, and won the point.

Still unsatisfied, I served again. "Maybe you could just call the school board and ask what to do in this situation."

"No, no, no," John said, annoyed that we were still playing. "It's fine. Getting up early is a small price to pay for being with you. I don't mind at all. As a matter of fact, I'm getting more sleep sleeping with you than I have in a year. Somehow you've cured the insomnia I've had since I quit drinking." I reluctantly put my racket down.

But still I could barely take it. What did he think, that the school board—which was, as he well knew, desperate for substitutes and especially ones who dared to go to South Central—would not allow for subs to have dates that ended in sleepovers? That would certainly be a surefire way of cutting down the people who'd fill in for sick teachers—leading to even more chaos in an already chaotic environment.

After several weeks of John's driving across the city at 4:30 A.M., I finally convinced him to call the motherfucking school board to ask what he should do if he was sleeping elsewhere. The answer? Drumroll, please: leave the new number on his outgoing message. It was no problem—no problem at all. *How sad it was*, I thought, *that he was so afraid*.

During this falling-in-love time, we had sex. We were never an I-can't-wait-to-fuck-you, fuck-each-other-all-the-time couple. But after that first crying sex, after I finally let myself fall in love with John, we'd have sex, maybe once or twice a week, sometimes less, once in a while more.

At the very beginning, I was daring. During one of our early hour-long phone conversations, I started to talk dirty on the phone and John was interested. He walked himself into his bathroom for privacy as I brought him to climax. I'd learned phone sex from Frankie, a guy I dated the summer before I moved back to L.A. One day he just started telling me things he'd like to do to me. I quickly took to being worked up and to working him up. (Before Frankie's introduction, I had thought phone sex was just for lonely, old, ugly perverts who had to call 800 numbers to get off.)

But I kept at playing the hot-for-sex sex-kitten. One day while John was on the phone with his roommate who was at work, I unzipped his pants and quickly got him interested. I sucked him and sucked him while he carried on his conversation and he even managed to come while he continued talking. He seemed to love it and I loved it that he loved it. I was proud, if not satisfied. I was still chasing after the high of Frankie's phone sex/Stuart's kinkiness, doing stuff to John that I hoped would turn us both on. And while John was responsive, it wasn't really something he craved or initiated.

Some nights, at the height of our we-can't-stand-to-be-away-from-each-other time, I'd pull up into his driveway and jump out as fast as I possibly could because I couldn't wait for his wide-open arms to hold me. We couldn't wait to jump in bed and sidle up to each other and wrap our bodies around each other and lie with our heads on our pillows, facing each other, just staring at each other, completely engrossed—and shocked and relieved that we had actually found each other. And sometimes, on one of those I-can't-wait-to-see-you nights, we'd sex.

One time John gently moved me on top of him. I was on my knees straddling him, hovering over him. And he traced my breasts very gently with his finger. I loved him moving me into the position he wanted and I loved him being slow and quiet.

And then there was the day fucking. Daytime worked well for us because we were full of energy. With the bright sunlight flooding my bedroom, we'd have a quick fuck in between the day's activities. Or sometimes, John would pull my pants down when I was lying on his living room sofa and give me head as I looked out the window at the neighbors passing by until I'd finally close my eyes in pleasure and come. That was fun, though one-sided.

On our first road trip to Mammoth, we talked about pulling off the highway to do stuff. Talking about it got us both so worked up that John told me to get off at the next exit, so he could give me head. We couldn't find a place where the car would have been hidden so we settled for a huge open field. I drove to the center of it and parked. I climbed halfway into the back seat and gazed out the rear window as John pulled my pants down. I quickly came, pulled up my pants, put my car in first gear, and was soon back on the highway. When we got to Mammoth, we fucked in the loft of the condo and John said he double came—he'd never felt anything like it.

And my personal favorite was one sunny afternoon, when I was lying facedown on my bed. John had me pinned in a way that I could barely move

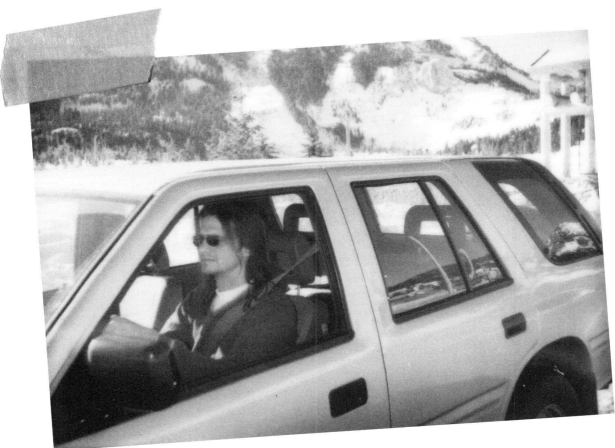

yet managed to dig my pelvis into the mattress, back and forth, back and forth. The restraint magnified my frustration, making my orgasm that much stronger.

We became roughly what I had always wanted: a normal in-love couple with a normal sex life.

Driving up to Mammoth, we got so turned on talking dirty that we pulled over in a field so John could give me head.

twenty-two

love, sex, and grandparents

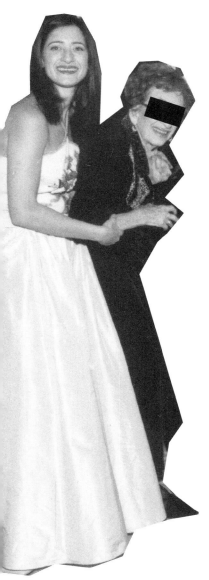

I had been hiding my prince from my family. But I knew the time to make the introductions was drawing near. I thought I'd practice giving the news by telling my dad's mom, Grandma Ruth, first. Not only was she less prim and proper than Grandmother Honey, I knew she wouldn't tell anyone, as she'd virtually stopped using her vocal cords in favor of pointing. After about a quarter second of a beat, however, she managed to eke out a gravelly, "What's his last name?" She was very feeble, but not out of it.

Disappointed by my answer, she grunted, "As long as you don't marry him."

Even though Grandma Ruth never went to synagogue, couldn't recite a blessing if you paid her, and liked Christmas far better than Hanukkah, she expressed her allegiance to her People by refusing to drive German cars and strongly disapproving if any of her children or grandchildren married a non-Jew. But she was open-minded and liberal on other fronts. Surprisingly for a woman of her generation, born in 1911, she wasn't anti-premarital sex. Every time I had ever told her I had broken up with someone (or more precisely that he had broken up with

Grandma Ruth had grown so feeble that she'd basically stopped talking. Therefore, I figured she'd make the perfect family member to practice breaking the news about my boyfriend on.

me), she would say it was because I'd slept with him too fast. At least she knew that I'd had sex.

On the other hand, my mother's parents, Grandpa Julius and Grandmother Honey—who were also, by the way, born in 1911—were totally against sex before marriage. This I learned one terribly uncomfortable morning at their breakfast table when I asked what I thought was a rather benign question: "Have you heard from Marney lately?"

My cousin Marney was living in Hawaii with her boyfriend Noah—a Jewish attorney who was born in Kansas City. My grandparents were Jews from Kansas City. I figured Noah would be my grandparents' wet dream. But I was wrong. They weren't so pleased with Marney and Noah. They weren't married. They were *living* together.

"Your grandpa and I do *not* believe in this pre-mar-i-tal sex," Grandmother matter-of-factly and slowly explained. As she carried on with her belief system, Grandpa ate his cereal and I cringed without looking up. While of course her views weren't so surprising, you should know that she absolutely loved *The People vs. Larry Flynt* and as a result was a huge Courtney Love fan. I wondered what went through an eighty-eight-year-old woman's mind when she watched a film about porn. Additionally, she had taken President Clinton's side in the Monica debacle. W*hat did people expect*, she rhetorically asked me, *for men not to cheat? A*nd *not to lie about it?* Hanging on her every word, I wished I had the chutzpah to ask her why she thought adultery was an inevitability for most men, even though I thought I knew. The big rumor in the family was that Grandpa had had a long-standing affair with his secretary. So while they were very high-and-mighty about premarital sex, they weren't so high-and-mighty about extramarital sex.

"Where should we go shopping today, Grandmother?" was my non sequitor response to her speech. I couldn't handle the conversation going any further in any direction.

I wasn't dying to introduce John to my parents either. I had never fully forgiven my mother for urging me to go on a blind date with a Jew when I was, for all she knew, happily committed to non-Jewish Auggie. John, on the other hand, was eager to meet everyone. Parents always loved him. "Bring it on!" he'd say. I wondered how badly my thinking they wouldn't approve made him feel.

Clearly the time had come to find a new therapist. And this time she had to already be married.

The moment I met Dr. Lynn Braun (DLB) in her chic, soothing, shades-of-sage office, I knew I'd found her. It was a relief to be back. I certainly couldn't negotiate a serious boyfriend and graduating from grad school with no moneymaking prospects all by myself.

twenty-three

outfits and tv shows

Every morning John drove his down-and-out Granada to South Central to be treated like shit by students who called him Mr. Beer, Mr. Queer, Hippie, and White Guy. But that was okay with him, he knew how to handle the enormous, intimidating sixteen- and seventeen-year-old gang-member kids—and he took some pride in that. He quickly realized that as their teacher for the day, he'd never be able to actually teach them anything. Rather, his job was to keep the peace. To that end, he managed to get the kids to draw pictures of him and write essays about what they thought his life was like. "Mr. Lehr sits in front of the TV and drinks beer," was the consensus. With the students occupied, he took advantage of the time and wrote dark, bizarre short films on his laptop.

On the rare occasion that he actually got an audition that he had a one-in-ten-thousand chance of getting, he wouldn't go in to sub that day, which meant his finances would be considerably more strained for the week. As much as I wanted to, I simply couldn't relate to how it felt to try to navigate his life. How was he so upbeat when he had student loans to pay off, credit-card debt to keep down, five grand to pay back to his friend who had covered his attorney fees when he was arrested for drunk driving (and charged with two felonies and two misdemeanors) plus rent, insurance, and dates with me to go on? I didn't know how he did it. I was just relieved that his arrest had led him to get sober and into therapy. I didn't need to be dating an alcoholic. On the contrary, I was thrilled to be dating someone in therapy, because I figured he was figuring out his tracks as well and maybe avoiding them with me.

In stark contrast to my struggling boyfriend, I was still in graduate school, living on more money than I should have had. My student-loan money kept coming in. Being a teacher's assistant at UCLA paid fairly well. And my parents still—though it was a source of constant heartache for all of us—paid my rent, car insurance, health insurance, dentist/doctor bills, and car repairs. I even had a cush part-time job working for a wealthy recently divorced woman who was shocked when her husband of twenty-eight years announced he was leaving her and was even more shocked when she found out that he was leaving her for his therapist (who well knew he was a multimillionaire). Though I was hired to teach her how to use her Macintosh, I ended up sorting through her lifetime of loose photos and spent months creating album after album of her former life. This all added up to an I'm-in-for-a-rude-awakening lifestyle of great clothes, expensive shoes, chic used furniture, good meals, and overpriced cocktails.

But it was more than in the back of my mind that it was going to quickly come to an end. School would soon be over and so would my teaching jobs. And I had long since glued my divorcée's last photo into an album. I managed to extend the life of my job by cleaning out the boxes from her old life that filled two spaces of her three-car garage, front to back, bottom to top. But that well was quickly running dry. What was I going to do with my life? How was I going to find a real job that would cover my expenses and pay insurance? My mother had clearly had it with me. This helping me out couldn't just continue indefinitely. How had the three years of school passed so quickly? Had I accomplished anything? I did my best to ignore the avalanche of reality that was heading my way while John toiled away in the avalanche of reality that had long since hit him.

Meanwhile, I had other work to do. I had a frog that had turned into a prince but still dressed like a frog. His closet was a disaster. I couldn't take the ninety-seven thousand oversize T-shirts on wire hangers. I couldn't bear his Dockers pants with pleats. No pleats. No Converse. No too-big-for-him T-shirts. I could only handle so much bad taste for so long.

Not wanting to overwhelm him, I introduced John to the concept of the white T-shirt. I explained that he would look so much better in a semi-fitted, plain crewneck T-shirt. He could wear it

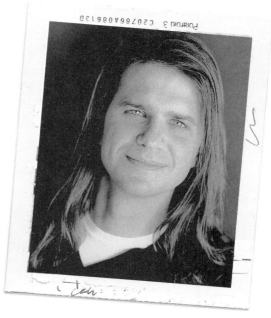

Ah, the difference a white T-shirt can make.

alone, under a button-down, or under a V-neck sweater. His big shirts, while they might tell the world he loves Metallica or remind him of some improv show he was in in Chicago, made him look like a scarecrow. Having already spent forty dollars on the used dresser I highly recommended he buy, John wasn't so amenable. Ahh yes, but did he know that a package of three was only eleven dollars on the Venice boardwalk? That's all I was asking. Just a single pack for eleven dollars. Still unsure, he dutifully followed his fashionable new love's fashion advice.

John quickly took to his new look. He wore his three white Ts three days in a row, but then had to switch to his oversize tents until laundry day rolled around eleven days later. How he loved those three days. When he lamented the situation, I made the mistake of suggesting he buy *another* pack. He got mad. Mad in a way I'd never seen before. I didn't know what to say.

Apparently my suggestion made him feel like my suggestions were never going to end.

"First a dresser for forty dollars, then T-shirts for eleven dollars, and now another eleven dollars! This is getting out of control. I can't spend my one day off shopping with money I don't even have. I've already lost a day's pay this week for a stupid audition that I tanked, why would I spend another eleven dollars? I have a closetful of clothes!" he said, his voice escalating with every word.

I felt terrible that I was so oblivious to his pressures. They were so hard to relate to, seeing that I had long since convinced myself that six hundred dollars was okay to spend on boots. (*They're classics! You'll wear them five days a week*, I'd tell myself, but then inevitably I'd love them a lot less by the next season.) At the same time, however, I wondered why he was complaining to me about not having enough white T-shirts in the first place if he was so goddamned happy with his closetful of clothes. Unfortunately, doing the laundry earlier than planned was also not an option and something else I shouldn't have suggested. He had so little time to himself, he just couldn't be running to the Laundromat every few days. He was a man of schedules. And he clung to them with his life. Laundry was done on Sundays every two weeks, period. Me, I didn't even own a calendar.

But soon he didn't like that he only liked how he looked three days out of every two weeks. So much so that without any prompting on my part, he went back to the boardwalk. Then he liked how he looked six days out of every two weeks. Building an arsenal of white T-shirts would take time and patience.

One day, I was surprised to see him looking so cute in dark Levi's. *Hey*, I thought, *maybe he does have some sense of style*. When I told him I loved the jeans, he said, "These? I was embarrassed to wear them in front of you, but everything else was dirty. They're a hand-me-down from Joey." Did he not realize his friend Joey was a shopaholic who always looked great? Disappointed but undeterred, I told John that I loved him in the jeans and that they'd look good with one of his white Ts. "And wait, what are these in the back of your closet?"

"Oh, those are just the old Kmart construction boots I wear camping."

"Well, they're great. Wear them with your dark Levi's and white T. And what about this gray sweater?"

"Lauren gave it to me for my birthday last year."

It seemed his friends were trying to give him hints, but had refrained from the straightforward talk he desperately needed.

At a party the following weekend, it was clear that everyone was surprised to see him looking so good. Virtually every friend commented— which made me feel both good and sad. It was so painfully obvious that people were happy to see him looking not ragged and like the decade since college hadn't passed. Jeans, a white T, construction boots, and a wool V-neck . . . et voilà, a man saved from himself.

Encouraged by my success, I bravely mentioned that I thought we should go through all the T-shirts hanging in the closet and weed some out. Despite the fact that he could admit that he didn't wear most of them, he didn't want to get rid of any.

"Maybe some other time," he said, clinging to what he had.

While a closetful of clothes made him feel less broke, I was desperate to prove that less was actually more. So one day, when he had to go over to his friend's for a few hours, I thought I'd show him what I meant. And just as I was hoisting an overloaded armful of oversize Ts onto the bed, John returned unexpectedly and opened the front door, where he had a clear view of what I was doing. He freaked out. Not so much angry as he was panicked, he screeched, "What are you doing?"

"I thought your Ts should be folded and put in your new used dresser. Pants and button-downs should be hung, not T-shirts. We can put in the shirts you love and wear most," I said as if I were going to let him wear them at all.

It took John a little hard-for-me-to-bear while to calm down. Once I

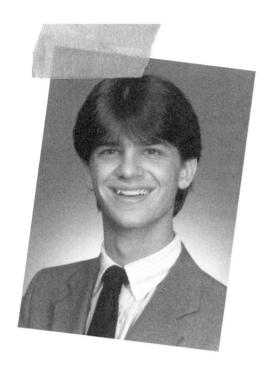

I was afraid that if John cut his hair he would revert to looking like the long-necked dork he was as a seventeen-year-old.

explained my system of piles—theater Ts, concert Ts, giveaways, must-keeps—he was up for changing his life. Soon he found himself in the garage getting boxes in which to store his sentimental favorites. On a roll, we moved on to shoes, jackets, and sweaters. Four hours later, we took everything he didn't want (or that I convinced him he didn't want) over to the Salvation Army.

He was starting to understand that he didn't need to look as broke as he was. His new look was doing wonders to mitigate his long hair and I was shocked when he said he was considering cutting it. Now, while I'd never dreamed I would be dating someone with long hair—a look I never even liked in the eighties—I was scared. I'd seen a photo of him the last time he had short hair and I didn't like what I'd seen. True, he'd been an awkward seventeen-year-old, but does one really grow into a too-long neck? Does an overly pronounced Adam's apple actually shrink? For some reason, I thought his hair hid these flaws. I was actually relieved when he told me he had to hold off for a while because there was a role on a new NBC sitcom that he actually had a good chance of getting, and it required long hair.

Back then I didn't have a clue how hard it was to be on a TV show—let alone understand how hard it was to get an agent in the first place. I didn't realize how few actors get to (A) audition for pilots for the casting director, (B) get called back to audition for the producers, (C) get called back again to audition for some more people though I'm not sure who, (D) get called back again to "go to network" before which all contract negotiations have to be made between the business-affairs department of the network, the actor's manager, the actor's agent, and the actor's attorney, and then finally

(E) actually get the part. And I also didn't know that once you had the part, you weren't guaranteed the part. If they didn't like you in the pilot, they could recast you. At any given moment you could be fired. So I didn't understand the gravity of what John was saying to me when he told me that he had a good chance of getting this part on a new sitcom that his friend Seth had created and that Seth had written a character named Junior—a long-haired eccentric who chose not to speak—with John in mind. If he didn't get the part, he was going to cut his hair.

We both hoped he'd get the job but didn't want to put too much hope into it.

With his new look and impending success, it was time to meet the family. If I waited until he'd gotten the job we hoped he'd get, it would be terrible. I wouldn't want John to think that I thought he was presentable only once NBC said he was.

twenty-four

the inevitable

I wasn't dying to call my mother to tell her I was bringing a date to Passover. I didn't want to hear her ask me any number of her super-earnest questions such as, "What are the qualities in John that you like the most?," which she inevitably would do during a cringe-filled lunch a month or so later. Her formal attempts to talk to my sister and me about our relationships, as if she were the kind of mother who had always talked to her children about their personal lives, made us both extremely uncomfortable. I forced myself to make the call. And to my relief the only question she had was the spelling of John's name. Was it J-O-H-N or Jonathan? She wanted to get it right for the place cards. She was happy to have him and looked forward to meeting him. Oh God.

Meanwhile, since I was a nervous wreck, I put my efforts into controlling the only thing I could: John's outfit. I wanted to do whatever I could to offset his long hair. My father was a very dapper dresser and my grandfather had been in the garment industry his entire life. The men in my family were more obsessed with clothes than the women—with the exception of me, of course.

After resurveying John's closet, I was reminded of how little I had to work with. In this case, less was actually nothing. I called Jason to see if we could borrow a jacket and told John that we had no choice but to buy some dress shoes. He had to have dress shoes—maroon Hush Puppies would never do. And John didn't balk because I guess he knew that for me this was not remotely an indulgence. And maybe he realized that it was about time he had a decent pair of dress shoes. I think he was relieved that finally someone was taking over—someone who truly cared and knew what the hell she was doing.

We met at Macy's and found a great pair for under a hundred dollars. He loved them and I loved them and loved that he loved them. Unfortunately, Jason's jacket was too big, so I decided he'd have to wear his own navy jacket even though the buttons were brass—we weren't Connecticut WASPs but it would do. Years ago, a friend had given him a blue striped shirt from Barneys. And even though the top button was cracked, it would have to do, too. On the way to pick John up, I passed a men's shop and pulled over to buy him some dress socks—I thought a nice pattern would make a better statement when he crossed his legs.

I also didn't love my outfit, so I stopped into a nearby store and purchased a new silk sweater set. I never felt as good as I did in something new and I was desperate for all the confidence my clothes could give me. Something new also guaranteed some ego stroking from my parents, who'd inevitably compliment me on how great I looked, what a nice this or that I had on. At those times they'd conveniently forget that I couldn't afford the purchase, that I'd charged it and was in over my head and we'd all have to deal with it in yet another finance fight that would end with me crying and my mom reluctantly writing what she hoped was one last check to pay off my Visa. It was a song and dance we all knew too well. I was obviously willing to put up with the fights, the resentment, the confusion, and the dysfunction to look good.

Almost thirty people were at the seder, so there were a lot of introductions to make and everyone was very friendly. We soon sat down, me nervously in between Grandmother Honey and John. Just before Grandpa started the service, Grandmother leaned across me. She looked John in the eyes and with a very warm smile said, "I'm very pleased to meet you." Pause. "Don't you think it is very difficult to raise children in a mixed religious household?"

How could she? I thought.

Holding her gaze, John smiled back and said, "Well, I'm very happy to meet you, too. And yes, I do agree, it can be very hard."

God, he's so good, I marveled to myself.

John loved the evening and everyone seemed to love John. By dessert he was surrounded by my family, answering questions, making everyone laugh, talking about his and my mother's hometown of Kansas City. He crossed his legs and flashed his new socks. I couldn't bear to watch it all go down, so I hung out in the living room. Periodically I'd peek in and find him laughing and holding everyone's attention. "He is so polite. So charming. What a great voice he had when reading his part of the Haggadah," more than a few people commented. None of these comments, however, came from my grandparents. They didn't say a word.

twenty-five

how to proceed?

Meanwhile, back at school, with just over a month to go before graduation, I started to feel very "fuck them!" Fuck all of the professors who thought I was a terrible person for writing about my feelings in my artwork. After their year of ignoring me didn't yield the results they hoped for, a couple of them resorted to literally imploring me not to publish my book. When I came across some well-timed advice to writers from author Tobias Wolff, I took it as my motto: "Don't be afraid of appearing angry, small-minded, obtuse, mean, immoral, amoral, calculating or anything else. Take no care for your dignity." *So what if people think I'm mean, calculating, and amoral I told myself. I'm being honest, which is more than I can say for anyone else. Being an artist is not a popularity contest.* Of course, my conclusion was easier to come to now that John loved me.

Meanwhile, I came up with the perfect idea for my MFA exhibition. I'd create an installation that looked like a table of books at Barnes & Noble that was featuring 78 *Drawings of My Face*. I became obsessed with designing and producing my book as if I was HarperCollins. I taught myself new tricks on Quark Xpress so I could format the book like a real book. I found a bookbinder downtown and a place to print the jacket I'd designed. Thousands of dollars later, my display was perfect.

Busying myself with the smallest details of my publishing project wasn't quite enough to distract me from my anxiety about the day that was fast approaching. What was I going to do when I graduated, when my student-loan money stopped pouring in, when I had to repay the loans? My divorcée no longer needed me. My teacher's-assistant jobs were up. My parents certainly wouldn't be happy to keep the faucet running postschool. I had no choice but to try to get famous—fast.

I asked my sister if she'd ask her old college boyfriend who was a big editor at a big publishing house if he'd read a chapter of 78 *Drawings* and recommend a few literary agents I could submit it to. She said yes, he then said yes, and soon I had a short list of four. And then, to my total thrill, I was signed by a New York literary agent. So while I was nervous about what to do next, I wasn't that nervous. I figured all I had to do was submit a proposal for the new book about sex that I'd started, sell it, write it, and bam—my life would be born. My plan of using my three graduate-school years to get my career going was actually working. I prematurely patted myself on my back.

Signing with my new agent gave me the courage to ask my parents to continue their thousand-dollars-a-month assistance. I needed some time to get on my feet, I explained. And I wasn't going to rely solely on the sale and subsequent success of my book, I was also developing my Celebration Book business. Celebration Books were private-edition, custom-made coffee-table books about a person's life. Over the years, I'd graduated from making a color-copied comb-bound book for Grandpa's eighty-fifth birthday to a two-hundred-page computer-designed book on my father's life. In between Grandmother got a booklet and my mother a magazine. My ideal clients would be wealthy people who already had everything money could buy, who would love a very personal gift. In a city teeming with rich people, I thought I could find my market. I was sure my parents, who had enjoyed the fruits of my labor, could see the potential for the business even if it did cater to a supersmall niche. And they did. They were cautiously optimistic and agreed to help with some start-up money.

Financial negotiations with my parents regarding our temporary arrangement were the smoothest ever because my new therapist, DLB, had strongly recommended they be done via fax and I followed her advice. The goal, according to the now Notorious DLB, was to make it as impersonal as possible. She had encouraged me to ask my parents to come up with a figure they felt 100 percent comfortable giving me, to ensure they wouldn't end up resenting me for giving it to me. If it was zero dollars, fine. Giving it serious thought, my parents told me that they felt comfortable helping me out for a finite period of time. I had nine months until the well ran dry. Nine months to finish and sell my book, or get my business up and running. Ideally, both. For the moment, I was relieved but I knew the clock was ticking.

twenty-six

motherfucking show business

Seven nerve-racking auditions later, John landed the job of playing Junior—the mute brother on NBC's new sitcom that would air between *Friends* and *Frasier*. This was "must-see" TV—the big time. Unlike virtually every pilot, this one had a guaranteed order of thirteen episodes. So if John could manage to keep his job through the making of the pilot, he wouldn't have to drive to South Central for a good long while. My parents— in a lovely gesture of support—wanted to take us out to celebrate.

This show, which warranted the most amount of money paid for a TV show in the history of TV at that time, was about a beautiful, blond, young, single mom who was taking care of all the men in her life—her son, her two brothers (one, a weird self-imposed mute, and the other, not so bright) and her bigoted father, an Archie Bunker wannabe. Would she ever have time for herself, time to pursue her dreams of becoming a nurse, let alone have time to go on a date?

John was excited, for obvious reasons. Not only would he instantly and finally be out of debt, but he now had a real chance at a career as an actor. Soon the world would know how funny he was. It was all very exciting. He met the cast and did all of the publicity photos. He worked with the PR department on his bio. He was even selected out of the cast of eight to go with the star and the man playing her father to the big press junket. *Wow*, he thought, I *really must have a good part in the show.* John's dressing room was big and comfortable. Rehearsals were going well. Everything was great, great, great.

The day came to shoot the pilot. While John was nervous, he wasn't nearly as nervous as he would have been had he any lines to deliver. As the brother who took a vow of silence for no apparent reason, he only had to make faces, point, nod, and walk. His dressing room, like those of all the actors, was filled with flowers and more flowers and gift baskets galore from his agents, from Warner Brothers, from NBC, from the star of the show and from the creator. "Welcome to the NBC family. Congratulations!" The production assistants were happy to get John anything he needed at any given second that he might need it. Altoids? Sure, I'll be right back. John had already started fantasizing about the new used car he would buy. It would have both an FM radio *and* an air conditioner.

Well, it turned out that more than a TV show was being made that night. Man wasn't landing on Mars and a peace treaty between Israel and Palestine wasn't being negotiated, but something equally important seemed to be taking place. This was NBC must-see TV in the making. There was nothing funny about making a comedy, and the throngs of security guards, executives, assistants, agents, managers, lawyers, and CEOs were proof of that.

On the set of the pilot, the president of the network felt sparks. The Beautiful Blond single mother and the guest star—the Latin Lover whom she didn't have time to date—had *Dharma and Greg* chemistry. The president had an idea. Let's scrap the entire concept of the show right now. Let's make it a show about the single mother ignoring her child, her family, and her ambitions. We'll hinge each episode on whether the Beautiful Blonde should or should not or should or should not or should or should not or should or should not or should or should not or should or should not date the Latin Lover. We'll keep America on pins and needles to see if this Beautiful

Blonde will ever find happiness with the handsome Latin Lover. Let's forget that we've spent a year developing this show, that we paid more money for the concept than we have for any other sitcom to date, that we told the creator we loved his idea and believed in him, that the creator had spent a year thinking about what he wanted to do with his show, that we've just spent months and hundreds of thousands casting and developing this show. Let's scrap everything. This is magic. As if he were a four-year-old little girl, the president was still seduced by Barbie and Ken.

So the family members who thought they were actually hired to be characters on a sitcom instantaneously became extremely well-paid extras. But it took John some time to realize what had happened. John thought for sure that his fairly-original-for-a-sitcom character would get to do some stuff—surely the comedy of a self-imposed mute was ripe for the picking.

Let me quickly tell you the weekly routine of making a sitcom—if you don't already know—so you'll be able to see more clearly how we let the show fuck up our lives in general and our sex life in particular.

Sitcoms are shot once a week. At around midnight, toward the end of "show night," a production assistant knocks on your dressing-room door and gives you—you being a regular cast member on the show who is not the Beautiful Blonde or the Latin Lover—an envelope. After your fifteen-plus-hour day, you open that envelope, take out the script of the next episode, and quickly flip to the second page. You focus your eyes on the little chart that tells you which scenes you will be in. Once in a blue moon you count all the way up to four. You'd be happy with four, but more often than not, you aren't happy. So then you (you not being the BB or the LL) flip open the script to those scenes you have and are either more depressed or less depressed based on the amount of lines—or moments, if you're a mute—you do or do not have. And after you've taken this all in, in less than thirty seconds, you tell your girlfriend that you think it's time to go home. You take her hand, very happy to have such a wonderful supportive girlfriend's hand to take, and you smile at everyone as you walk out of the soundstage, saying "good night, good show" to the other actors, and "good night, thank you for everything" to the wardrobe people, the makeup people, the grips, and the security guards—all of whom think you are particularly nice and what a cute couple you and your girlfriend make and how great it is for you that you've gotten your big break because clearly—based on the piece-of-shit car you're getting into—you desperately needed it.

You go to bed, wake up the next morning, read the whole script, and work on your tiny bits so that you can do your best at the "table read" later that day. If you do a great job raising your eyebrows in a funny way, maybe, just maybe, they'll give you a few more bits.

The room at the table read is full of all the writers who are anxious to see what you'll do with their words and to see how their script flies with all of the executives who are jam-packed in the room. Standing about are the show's execs, the production company's execs, the network's execs, and all of their assistants. And when you walk into this room, everyone smiles at you and says, "Great show last night." And then the room is quiet and the brain surgery begins.

And then based on these brilliant readings (which you had little time to work on because you were shooting the show until one in the morning), the writers go back to their writers' room and figure out how to make the script tighter and funnier. And you go home and work on your script because you have rehearsal the next morning, but you don't work too hard because you know that at seven o'clock in the morning a revised—more than likely heavily revised—script will be delivered to your door, copied onto pink paper to indicate that it is the second draft.

And then at seven o'clock you wake up and go to the door and open that envelope and look at that chart on the first page to see if they liked you, as evidenced by whether you have more scenes or less than you had at the table read. And then you flip to your scenes to see if you have more lines or less—or moments, if you are a mute. If you have less, you might start blaming yourself for doing a bad read yesterday—even though you only nod and make faces. If you have more, you might think that it is a result of your performance—which most of the time it is not. If you continually have stuff cut, you might start worrying that you are going to be fired, that you'll be broke and doomed to a life of failure, that all of your friends will think you're a loser. Your head might start to spin, obsessing on all of these negative thoughts. And then regardless of how you really feel, you arrive on the set full of smiles and hugs because after all you are grateful for your job, and you do like these people and you want desperately for them to like you. Maybe next week you'll be featured in an episode. Meanwhile it's not so bad getting paid a lot of money to sit in your dressing room all day. All your hopes are pinned on next week's script.

And then you go home and work a little on your bits and then you go to sleep, and in the morning the same thing . . . another envelope with a script now copied onto mint green paper has landed on your doorstep. And you go through the same shenanigans as you did the day before. And then the next day you go through the same routine again. And then one more day of it. If your character just happens to be a self-imposed mute, it's not so hard to learn your new gestures, moments, or actions every day. The challenge is remembering all of the marks you have to hit for the camera. For a single scene you might have to hit twenty-five different marks.

Finally, on show night, you tape the show live in front of an audience of mainly tourists. All of the writers watch the show, listen to the audience response, and try to come up with newer funnier lines (or bits) for you on the spot.

And John had a lot of feelings about all this that he had a hard time expressing—such as fear and anger. Fear of losing his job and anger that his friend Seth, the creator of the show, wasn't the kind of guy who could fight for what he wanted, anger that his friend couldn't manage to write him more clever stuff, anger that his friend would let them write him out of the scripts almost completely and not give John the courtesy of an explanation, fear of not ever getting his big chance, frustration at the stupidity of it all anyway, angry that he could care so much about having more lines on such a stupid show, and then rage at being so fucking powerless. But it was, he'd remind himself, better than substitute teaching in South Central, hoping that it would help those intense feelings feel less intense. After all, what right did he have to those feelings when his salary was so high and the opportunity was so potentially great? Trying to remain positive, John tried not to think about all of the sitcom actors he watched growing up whom he'd never seen work again.

Every morning, as soon as the alarm went off, I prayed that the new script that I knew was leaning against the front door of our building would give John more to do—my happiness (meaning the amount of attention, affection, and sex John would give me) depended on it. I had no understanding of the concept that I could be happy if John was unhappy. I was always upset that he was upset and I was extra upset when he took his upset out on me.

On a typical morning when the alarm would go off, I'd fly downstairs to pick up the envelope. I'd open it and look at the front page to see what my week would be like. Going back up in the elevator, I'd nervously flip through the pages to see how much John had to do. And then I'd open the door to the apartment and reluctantly hand it to him, unable to stave off the inevitable. Then he'd flip through and feel lots of feelings and I'd feel different feelings watching him feel those feelings—feelings like anger at him for letting the stupid show upset him so much, anger at his friend for not giving him more to do, and fear of how his mood was going to affect our relationship.

Desperate to come up with something that would make our lives better, I thought exercise would help John relieve stress. Similarly desperate, he was amenable. So three mornings a week, we'd put on our hiking outfits and I'd drive us over to Runyon Canyon while he sat next to me reading the script changes, trying to figure out how he could make something of his little bone. And he'd work so hard on his little bone, despite being so upset that that was all he had to work on. If I said something while he was figuring out a funny way to do his bone, he'd bark at me. He was busy, he couldn't be talked to. He had a bone to attend to. And I'd feel hurt and want to tell him to fuck off, but at the same time I knew that a fight would further distract him from working and that would make him even more mad at me. I felt trapped.

And then he'd go to work, arriving early—always early. He never wanted to be the one to cause problems. (Often I'd wish he was more like Evan. When I was dating the ESCBB and he was on a TV show, he was always late. I can't tell you how many times we'd sleep through his alarm only to get a call from the line producer that he had better hurry up and get over to the lot. Evan had a more they-should-be-happy-to-have-me-on-their-stupid-sitcom attitude. I don't know where he got it, and sometimes it was too much, but God, I wished John had some.) Everyone at work absolutely loved John, but it didn't get him more of a part.

And me, well, I'd go to therapy and tell the Notorious DLB how John was getting mad at me for just talking at the wrong time. It's like he thought anything I did could fuck up his concentration and then he'd fuck up his part and then he wouldn't get more to do and then he wouldn't get to be funny on TV and therefore wouldn't get any more work. He'd snap at me with the force of his entire career on the line. And I'd apologize because how could I understand the pressure he was under?

Inevitably DLB would make me see how clearly wrong it was that John took his frustrations out on me. Driving home, I'd get madder and madder by the traffic light. As soon as John would come home from his day—uneventful except for the feelings he was feeling in his new tiny dressing room that was a trailer outside of the soundstage—he was able to tell that there was a lot wrong just by looking at my enraged face that could never hide how I was feeling even if I tried. The second I saw him, I'd just blurt out what I wasn't going to take from him anymore. He couldn't talk to me the way he did or be mad at me for things I didn't do. It wasn't my fault they changed the script every day and it wasn't my fault they'd changed the show and it wasn't my fault they didn't give him more to do.

I had no idea how to present my feelings in a way that was conducive to actually having them (A) heard and (B) understood. And so, in about five seconds we'd be fighting. He'd become defensive and I'd become enraged that he was explaining away his behavior. I would get so mad I'd slap my hands together really hard or hit my leg. And I would just scream and scream, louder and louder, until he couldn't take it. Sometimes he'd just walk out the door, leaving me in tears.

And sometimes when he came back we'd try to talk about what happened. Sometimes we'd make progress, though evidently not enough because inevitably just around 11 P.M. the tension would swell again. I wouldn't want to go to bed without resolving everything. I'd be ready to go at it—again. And he'd be appalled that I'd have the nerve to fight right when it was bedtime. He had to work tomorrow. And I'd be furious because I knew he had so little to do at work and wasn't our relationship important enough for us to work things out? "Fine," I'd often say, "I'll be sleeping on the sofa." And off I went—at once eager to be away from him and aware that my leaving would get to him.

"Please come back to bed, honey," he'd beg, exhausted and anxious.

Sometimes I would, sometimes I wouldn't. Sometimes it was such a relief to be out there in the living room not having to feel so many intense feelings about the guy next to me. I wanted him to love me with the love and attention he used to. I wanted to remain lovable. Sometimes the fights would get so bad I'd forgo our sofa for my friend Jason's sofa.

Inevitably, the next day we'd have a serious talk in the living room. Facing each other in chairs on opposite sides of the coffee table, we'd both steel ourselves for the uncomfortable exchange that lay before us. We'd make our best efforts to calmly talk about what had happened, but—unable to help ourselves—we'd continuously and indignantly interrupt, interject, and correct. Neither of us would let the other make it through an entire thought. Both of us wanted to be heard, neither of us knew how to listen.

During one of these living-room sit-downs, John remarked how he noticed that things would be fine between us, or relatively fine, and then I'd go to therapy and I'd come home enraged and then we'd fight. He said that while he did want to hear what I had to say and he was glad that I went to therapy, he didn't think it was healthy or helpful for us to talk about what the Notorious DLB and I had talked about the same day of my therapy. John said my newly stoked anger made a constructive conversation impossible. And he wanted me to keep in mind that DLB only heard my side. So I agreed to wait twenty-four hours to evaluate how I felt and what I thought, and then if I wanted to have a discussion, I would ask him when a good time was. I promised to try not to erupt out of nowhere. With this agreement, we made up. John asked me if I wanted a hug and sheepishly I nodded. He took a step toward me and then I took one toward him and soon I found myself in his arms just where I wanted to be, upset by the route that I had to take to get there.

Sex as a form of making up wasn't our style—at all, ever. As a matter of fact, our sex life had diminished to virtually nothing since the stupid show started. He was either too upset or too busy to do it. I was desperate for the attention and he knew it but avoided the subject and me—when we were alone together—like the plague. But when others were around, he was more affectionate. While I was happy to take what I could get, I wanted more than he was offering.

Because I didn't cook and because John worked late, more often than not we found ourselves out to dinner. John would pick up the tab, seeing that he was making more in a week than I'd make in the year. It wasn't something we discussed. It's just something that happened. And when we were out, he'd let me stick my hand down the back of his pants and squeeze his gorgeous ass, and he'd put his arm around me and you'd think we were as happy as could be. And for a decent amount of time during the course of a week, we actually did okay. But when we'd get home, I'd wonder where the loving went. I'd lie in bed hoping holdings and kisses would come, but they wouldn't.

DLB explained to me, in one of my many I-don't-know-what-to-do-am-frustrated-as-hell-because-we-aren't-having-sex therapy sessions, that sometimes when men are frustrated with their careers, they respond in one of two ways: they either have more sex or less/bordering on none at all. In the case of the former, she said it was because the men find warmth and strength and maybe even power and control (in positive ways) in their relationship. But in the case of the latter—which is what she suspected was happening with John—he wasn't feeling good about himself or his career, so he wasn't feeling sexual. I was furious at NBC for ruining my sex life.

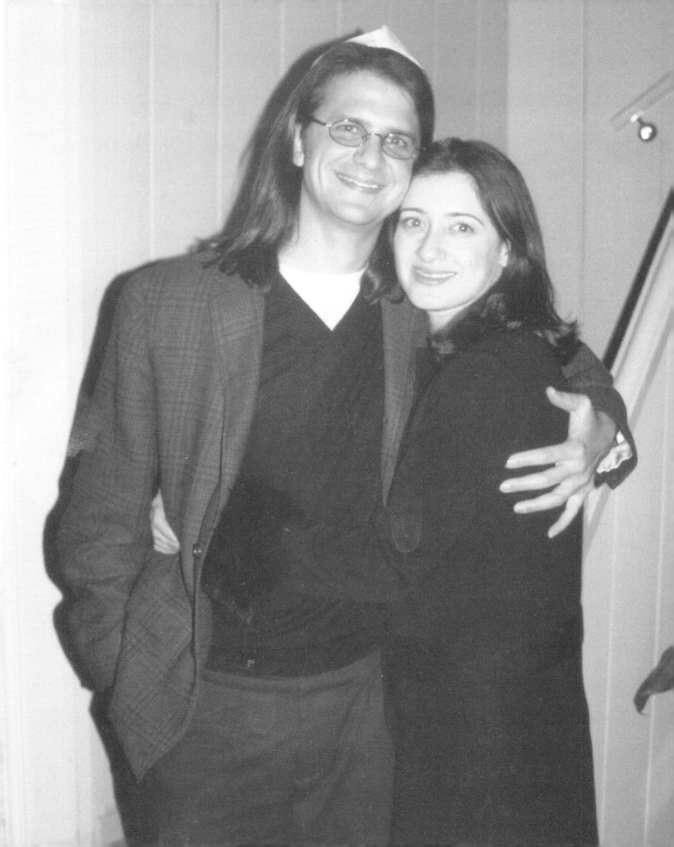

twenty-seven
motherfucking rabbi

John told me that he wanted us to take an introduction to Judaism course (i.e., a class created for those who want to convert). We weren't engaged. I didn't feel close to getting engaged. We weren't living together! We weren't even having sex. Why the hell would we take that kind of class?

"Honey, I'm not in any way saying I want to convert. It's just that Judaism is obviously such a big part of your family's life. I want to learn more about it. And that way, if we ever do get married, I will be educated and informed and will be able to tell your parents and grandparents, with respect, why I'm *not* converting."

Who could argue with that? But my goodness, he was planning ahead. Marriage? Me, married?

Though I was twenty-nine years old, I thought marriage was for adults. And I didn't feel like I was getting any closer to being one—except chronologically. To make my aging-but-not-successful self feel better, I'd replay the being-thirty-today-is-like-being-twenty-four-twenty-years-ago-I-have-plenty-of-time speech over and over again. I thought that being a wife meant I definitely had to be responsible and have a career—or a steady job—and be able to pay for my health insurance, car insurance, and rent without the help of my parents. I

In addition to white T-shirts and V-neck sweaters, John found himself sporting a *kepa* on Jewish holidays. And now he wanted to know why he wore it.

wanted to do those unimaginable things well before I got married. I didn't want to go from being dependent on my parents to being dependent on my husband. That would be so 1950s of me, and even though my parents were still helping me out (a lot), I somehow was able to still see myself as a thoroughly modern feminist. I saw my parents as investors. All businesses needed capital. Me, I was writing my book and I was working on my Celebration Books business by writing cover letters to party planners, putting together packages of my samples, photographing my work, designing a website and a brochure, and making press kits. I even had a booth at two wedding fairs that resulted in one real bona fide job. Like most new businesses, I was losing money before I was making it.

So before I could imagine being a wife, I had to be able to imagine being independent and I couldn't quite imagine what it would be like—what an independent Jennifer would look like, act like, live like. I figured I'd give up buying all of my chic clothes, actually balance my checkbook instead of periodically calling in for an account balance, eat all meals at home, and work for someone whom I would eventually resent. Imagining financial independence *and* being a wife was just out of my realm. *One major/life-altering thing at a time*, I thought.

The only "discussions" John and I had on the subject of marriage were my soapbox rants about how absurd I thought so many of the American rituals that preceded marriage were. Just so he knew, I had no interest in being proposed to. The stupid diamond-in-the-champagne-glass, ring-around-a-puppy's-collar, surprise-on-the-pillow, romantic-comedy variety of making the most serious decision in one's life astounded me. Wasn't it so obvious that marriage was something that should be discussed and decided together? I hated all of the stories I'd heard of the girl just waiting and waiting and waiting to be asked and the guy feeling pressured into it. And I hated the bullshit game a couple played when both knew they wanted to spend the rest of their lives with each other but the woman had to anxiously wait to be taken off guard and the man had to obsess over how, when, and where and to guess what kind of ring the woman would love to wear every single day of their forever. I hated the idea that often the groom-to-be's entire family and slew of friends knew his soon-to-be fiancée's fate before she did. What was romantic about that? I hated that only the woman received an engagement present that showed the world she was taken. I hated that only women had bridal showers. John was the cook between us, surely he should be the one to open up the typical pots-and-pans shower gifts. Those were the type of things I'd carry on and pontificate about. They were easier to deal with than the question "Why get married?"

Fortunately, John was in total agreement with me. We decided that at some time in the future—hopefully at a time when we weren't fighting so much and were sexing more—when we were ready to think seriously about marriage, we would make plans to go out to dinner and discuss it. Meanwhile, we enrolled in an introduction-to-Judaism course. John wanted to keep it between us until we'd completed the course, which was fine by me. I didn't want my family getting the wrong idea. We were not engaged and he was not becoming a Jew.

However, almost everyone in the class was engaged and converting. And in most cases, it was the man who was Jewish and his fiancée who was there to convert in time for their quickly approaching nuptials. Even though only one person in each couple was converting, in most cases both attended the class. (It was the most gorgeous girls with the biggest rings on their fingers who came alone.) As a matter of fact, in a class of sixty, Robert and Heidi were the only female-Jew, male-non-Jew couple there. Robert and Heidi had already been married for two years. They were considering having children soon and wanted to deal with the religion issue seeing that he still had an affinity for a Christmas tree.

We didn't quite have that problem because John grew up celebrating both Christmas and Hanukkah—and had a beautiful menorah to prove it. His mom was raised a Methodist and his father a Catholic—two religions that didn't like their kind marrying any other kind. So when his parents married, they denounced their religions, decided they were atheists, and joined the Unitarian church, which welcomed those of all faiths and faithlessness. The Unitarian church was more about community and taking the best of all religions. For instance, in the spring they acknowledged Easter, Passover, and the spring solstice, because they were all celebrations of rebirth. Despite all of these festivities, however, the only religious belief John inherited from his parents was their lack thereof. Like his parents, John considered himself an atheist until he started to read *For Those Who Can't Believe* by Rabbi Harold Schulweiss. My sister had recommended the book after John was blown away by his sermon at our Yom Kippur services.

Reading the book, John realized he wasn't really an atheist but rather an agnostic. After all, how could he be so certain that God did not exist? He was also surprised to learn that you could be Jewish and still question the existence of God. As a matter of fact, Judaism welcomed questioning God. Rabbi Schulweiss had certainly piqued his interest.

Our teacher was Rabbi Aaron Steinberg, who wanted to be called Rabbi, or Rabbi Steinberg, but never Rabbi Aaron. Rather proudly, in his introductory remarks, Rabbi Aaron told the class that many don't pass the first time around. As a matter of fact, only nine did in the last group. He was opening his class full of anxious, non-Jewish, soon-to-wed women with a threat. I didn't like this guy from the first twenty seconds of him.

Rabbi Aaron went on to explain that this class was just like any other college course, that it was an introduction to Judaism from historical, religious, and cultural perspectives and that anyone could certainly take it just as they would any other religion course at a liberal arts college. As a matter of fact, he explained, they offered college credit, if anyone was interested. I'm not sure who he thought he was kidding, but not one person in the class was there to just learn about Judaism as if they were taking a UCLA extension class in Renaissance art. Most of the women were there because they were engaged to Jewish men who wanted Jewish wives even though they themselves were nonpracticing Jews. When pressed as to why it was so important for their fiancées to convert, many of these men said they just couldn't handle being responsible for ending a lineage. Who were they to further diminish the population of the Jewish people—a people who had been perpetually persecuted for thousands of years, who had struggled and suffered so much to keep the faith alive?

The sitcom John was on had just aired a month earlier, so most people talked to him with an I'm-trying-not-to-be-excited-he's-in-my-class reverence. The most starstruck, however, was Rabbi Aaron, who loved that he had an actor on must-see TV in his class. He often asked John how the show was going and bragged about what other actors had taken his class. As a matter of fact, John was the only person in our class he knew by name.

Rabbi Aaron preyed on the weak. He seemed to take a perverse pleasure in making vulnerable brides-to-be cry. He thought nothing of telling a student who had suffered through him and his class for six months that she should take it again because she wasn't serious enough. Even though she'd done all the homework, studied for the tests, attended synagogue, practiced being kosher, and sung the songs, she was stupid enough to admit she had some questions, or to answer the questions on his test from her point of view and not his. After all, according to Rabbi Aaron, there was only one thing Rosh Hashanah was about and only a few specific words that one should use to describe it—those being his. If you didn't use his language and say exactly what he had written down on the study sheet, then he was sorry but you'd have to take that part of the test again. He was so beyond dumb that he thought making adults memorize his words showed that they had learned something, beyond learning that he didn't want them to think for themselves.

When I'd report his outrageous behavior to the Notorious DLB—floored that this was how Judaism was being taught—she said, prefacing it with her usual "it-would-be-malpractice-for-me-to-diagnose-him-without-meeting-him" disclaimer, he was a clinical narcissist, someone who was incapable of seeing beyond himself.

During the breaks, I'd hang out at the vending machines and commiserate with my classmates about Rabbi Aaron. Each anecdote they shared made my blood boil. I would try to get them to see that they didn't have to tell Rabbi Aaron everything. It wasn't necessary to confess that during their required week of being kosher, they had an Altoid because they didn't realize it wasn't kosher. That way the rabbi wouldn't tell them that he was sorry, but the week didn't count. That they had to start all over again. Rabbi Aaron took advantage of their need-to-be-Jewish-by-X-date situations. He basked in his power.

Rabbi Aaron didn't like to wait until you finished your question before he began to answer it because he couldn't give a shit why you were asking what you were asking. He didn't care what concepts you were struggling with. He was only interested in telling you that he had an answer for your question and that his answer was *the* answer to have even though he had just explained that one of the great things about Judaism is that it welcomes questions and is open to interpretation and that interpretations have evolved over the centuries. Just don't ask and interpret on his class time. Second-guess God, but not him.

Well, me, I second-guessed the fuck out of him every chance I got. After he was good and done giving his lecture (never interrupt him with a question, write it down and ask at the end when only five minutes remain), my hand always flew up. When called on, I'd point out contradictions he'd made or underline for the class yet another of his covertly sexist comments. He was infuriating, illogical, and smug and I wanted the class to know that they didn't have to take what he said at face value even if they weren't already Jewish. John couldn't take my behavior. When he'd see my hand go up, he'd beg me with his eyes to put it down. After a while, he asked me to please not try to pick fights with the rabbi. Yes, he totally agreed with me, the guy was a putz and a terrible representative of Judaism, especially to people who are considering converting, but he didn't want me to piss the rabbi off. He didn't want me to ruin his chances of passing the class.

I couldn't believe John was saying this, that he was so afraid of this narcissistic asshole. Rabbi Aaron had gotten John, too! The class needed to see that someone could stand up to him, that someone could question his interpretations. And I'd appointed myself that person. And John didn't think that I needed to be that person. I wasn't an elected union representative. John tried to explain to me that he, along with all of the other people, needed to pass this class. He had no desire to take it again. (Passing doesn't mean you've converted, it just means you are eligible to convert. And he wanted to keep his options open.)

I was furious at John for being intimidated by this loser. The last thing he should be concerned about was the rabbi not passing him just because I—a separate human being from John—stood up to him. And couldn't John see that if for some reason that actually happened, we could easily go above the rabbi's head? John was the best student in the class. Did he really think that Rabbi Aaron wouldn't pass him because his girlfriend had put him on the spot a few times?

John said that I had nothing to lose. I was already Jewish. Couldn't I please respect his request? He just wanted to get out of the class what he could and leave the rest. And he wanted a girlfriend who supported him, not one who worked against him. Even John, however, had a threshold. John insisted that we leave exactly at one o'clock sharp, whether or not the rabbi was finished with his lecture (which he never was). Rabbi Aaron got very perturbed if people arrived late, but he thought nothing of going forty-five minutes over.

But the strict one-o'clock departure wasn't enough of a fuck-you-Rabbi-Aaron for me. I didn't like John telling me what I should or shouldn't say to the rabbi. John thought I had no idea how it felt to really want something or need it and to be afraid that it would be taken away unfairly. And he resented me not only for not knowing how that might feel (meaning he resented me for being as confident as I was) but also for not respecting his feelings, for not respecting that he had a number of experiences in his life that led him to feel the valid way he felt.

On any given Sunday drive home from Rabbi Aaron's class, we'd fight.

Sometimes we'd fight because John couldn't believe I cared more about asking my question and attempting to humiliate the rabbi than I did about his feelings. Hadn't he asked me nicely not to push everything? And I'd be incredulous. I had a legitimate problem with the way Rabbi Aaron explained some sexist ritual and didn't think I should have to not speak up because my (wimpy) boyfriend was afraid it would affect his grade. And the fact that we hadn't eaten yet would further fuck us both over. We'd both be hypoglying, which dramatically affected our ability to think straight and fight fair. We'd come home hungry, angry, exhausted, and unglued. It wasn't uncommon for me to start crying hysterically only to have John resent me for trying to manipulate him with my tears. He couldn't stand it when I cried. "Just stop the crying," he'd demand. And when I couldn't control myself on command, he'd walk out the door exasperated. He couldn't send me to my room, but he could leave me in it. If I was going to cry, I'd have to do it alone. Having sex got further away from us by the Sunday.

Now not only did John have his script to obsess over and his busy TV-show schedule to keep, he had tons of Jewish books to read and funny-looking letters to memorize. He was less available than ever. This great thing he was doing for our relationship didn't seem so great to me. Whenever we'd tell a friend John was taking the class, they'd say, "Oh, he must love you sooooo much." And I'd think, *Well, I'd be happier if he showed his love by lying in bed cuddling and sexing me—not kissing ass to some narcissistic rabbi in his effort to kiss my family's ass.* I wanted my ass kissed—literally.

But I had to admit that there were some great things about taking the class together. We liked the readings. We did enjoy Shabbat dinner. We enjoyed going to synagogue. We liked singing the prayers. And we were friendly with some of our classmates. I couldn't help but enjoy learning more about my religion and culture even though it was from a rabbi I hated. And believe me, I hated hating a rabbi.

twenty-eight

motherfucking propecia

Meanwhile we wondered if it wasn't the Propecia John was taking that was to blame for his
seriously diminished interest in screwing. His
hair had undeniably started to thin all over, so the
minute he got the sitcom—which meant his SAG insurance had kicked in again—he got the sixty-nine-dollars-
a-month prescription. He was told that sometimes
Propecia just staved off any more hair loss and sometimes it actually regrew hair. He'd know which category
he fell into in about three months. The literature also
warned him of a potential side effect: a decreased libido.
However, the label said, that occurred in less than 3 percent of the users. While we waited for results, the hair-
stylists on the sitcom used dark powder on his scalp so
that it didn't shine through so much. Nothing is worse
than thin long hair.

The drug also came with the warning that a pregnant
woman should not touch a pill lest she expose her baby
to the possibility of birth defects. John was very paranoid
about this and decided he would never even touch the
pills himself. Each night he'd spill a pill onto the bottle
cap and then pop it into his mouth. I didn't know why he
was so paranoid—if we weren't screwing there wasn't a
chance I'd get pregnant. And besides, I was probably a

good solid five to ten years away from having a baby, should I ever decide to have one in the first place. John said he was practicing. He planned to take the drug for a long time because if he stopped, all of the hair he'd gained would fall out. He wanted his procedure to be a habit so he'd never endanger our unborn child. I couldn't imagine thinking that far ahead—particularly for a relationship that lacked a decent sex life. John was clearly more of an optimist than I was.

I asked DLB what she thought about the Propecia. I was at once hoping it was the cause of our problem because the puzzle would then be solved—and praying that it wasn't because I didn't want us to have to choose between sex and a bald head. I wasn't dying to have a bald boyfriend, and he wasn't dying to be a bald boyfriend.

DLB asked me if John had erections. Yes. I felt/saw it erect in the mornings. Taking it as a sign of interest, I'd touch it with intent to suck, but he wasn't interested. Mornings weren't a good time to screw for him, he was just waking up. He explained to me that his hard dick was not a sign of arousal, it just meant he had to pee. I'd never heard that before. Based on his penis's ability to be erect, DLB said she didn't think the Propecia was the problem, but added that she wasn't a medical doctor and that it was important to rule out any physical problems first. She suggested I encourage John to be checked out by a urologist.

He was surprisingly up for it, but I had to be patient. First he had to get a referral. Then he had to find a time, which wasn't easy when he worked five days a week. He had to wait for a hiatus week. I felt like the little girl in *Charlie and the Chocolate Factory* who wanted to try the unperfected gum ball that tasted like an entire meal NOW. I wanted to find out if Propecia was ruining my sex life NOW.

twenty-nine

motherfucking purse

Now that John was a successful TV actor making good money, he wanted to take us on a romantic getaway for Thanksgiving. (I was semisurprised that he was so willing to spring for the vacation, seeing that it took him two and a half months to decide if he should or shouldn't, should or shouldn't buy the ninety-nine-dollar corduroy jacket that he loved from the J.Crew catalog. After a good solid month of thinking about it, he finally okay'd the purchase only to tell me to hang up with the J.Crew operator mid-order. He needed more time to think about it.) John thought a drive up the coast would be nice—we could stay in Big Sur and then visit his brother, Steve, and his wife, Grace, in San Jose. I made the reservations.

We got a little cabin surrounded by redwoods. We hiked in the forest, walked on the beach, watched the sun set, and ate gourmet dinners. And finally, we did it. However, the sex under the cozy eiderdown in the charming cabin in the romantic woods wasn't what I'd wanted it to be. Yes, I rocked on top of John with his penis inside me. It's true he told me he loved me. I did come. And so did he. *What more could I ask for?* I asked myself. But the whole time we were doing it, I was analyzing it. Did he really love me or did he just feel like he should say he loved me

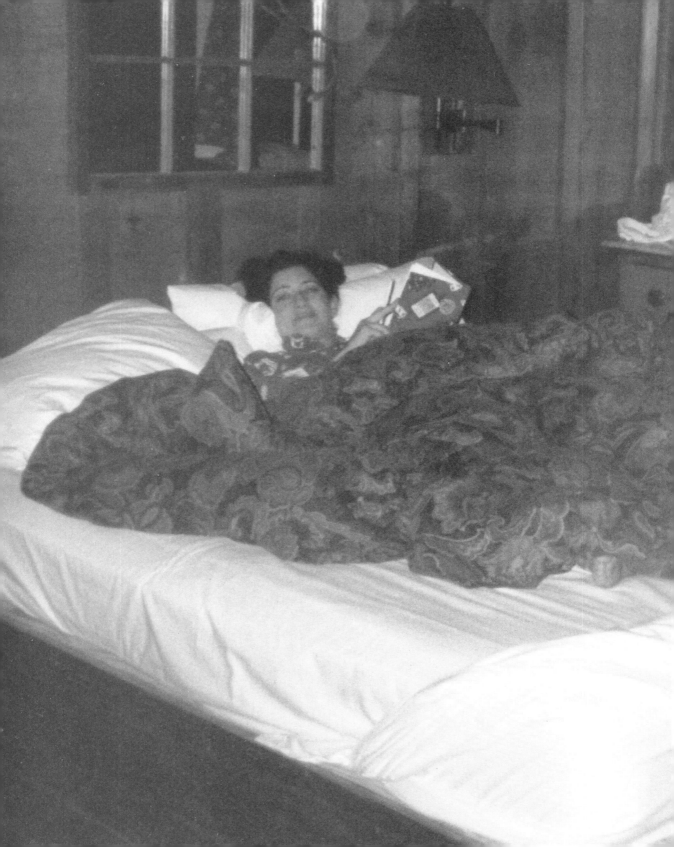

while fucking me in this romantic setting? If he did love me, wouldn't he have spent more time loving me before fucking me? Was he only sexing because he thought he should be sexing because we were on vacation and hadn't sexed for so long?

After a few semiperfect days in Big Sur, we left for San Jose. Unfortunately his brother, Steve, had a very troubled cat named Bubbles that hated everyone in the whole world—especially Steve's wife, Grace. Last time John visited his brother, Bubbles had peed on his duffel bag, so this time after we arrived, we made sure we put all of our luggage in the guest-room closet and kept the door shut. After our Yahtzee-filled visit, we drove to San Francisco, where we planned to spend the day doing nothing other than stroll around the city holding hands.

We found a parking garage near the water. I parked the car, and while John got out I looked in the backseat for my purse. *Wait, where is it*? I didn't say anything yet because I knew John couldn't take it when I lost shit. It wasn't unusual for me to panic for a moment when I couldn't find something, only to find it a minute later. But that moment of panic always drove John crazy. He always thought (and who could blame him?) that my purse, or wallet, or keys, or glasses were actually missing and that it was a huge tragedy. He couldn't imagine ever misplacing something. Who could be so irresponsible to lose their wallet? Wouldn't that just ruin your life?

"Let's go, honey," John said, ready to leave the garage.

"One second, ummm . . ." I said, stalling.

"What is it?" he asked.

"Ummm, I can't, well, umm, one second, let me just open the back up"—rummage rummage—"fuck"—rummage rummage . . .

"What is it, Jennifer?"

"Ummmm, well, I can't find, shit fuck, I guess I left my purse somewhere . . ." I forced myself to say as I scrambled to find my cell phone and the number to the inn in Big Sur. The reception sucked, but the person at the inn managed to make out what I was saying and could I hold on, and

Me in our cozy bed in our charming cabin on our romantic weekend in Big Sur, where we finally did what we hadn't done in a long time.

sorry, no, they haven't found anything, and yes, they'll call if they do, and John was just beside himself now, spitting with rage.

"What are your plans now?" John screamed. "What are you going to do without any money? How can you just lose things all the fucking time? How do you expect to get your car out of the garage? Who's going to pay for it? I am, right? You have no fucking idea how your carelessness affects others. How dare you waste the time of the poor staff at the Big Sur Inn over your stupidity! Those poor maids shouldn't have to stop what they are doing to look for something that isn't even there. How dare you think wasting other people's time isn't a big deal. This is bullshit!"

Panicked and frightened, I called John's brother, who confirmed that my purse was in the back of the closet where I had to fucking put it to keep it away from the stupid fucking bitch of a cat. Steven said it was no prob-lem . . . he'd FedEx it to me. I'd have it by the time I got home. John didn't give a shit that it had been found. His day, his vacation, was already totally ruined by his careless, someone-always-bails-her-out, doesn't-know-the-value-of-a-dollar, irresponsible, spoiled girlfriend. His brother shouldn't have to go to FedEx because I was so out of it.

I was in tears because he was so angry and he was furious that I had the nerve to cry when I was the one that had fucked things up. How dare I cry? I'd fucked up and now I had the nerve to cry to make him feel sorry for me? Now it was going to be about him yelling at me and not me being a fuckup? He wasn't going to fall for that shit. I had fucked up his first nice vacation in his life that he'd worked so hard for the last ten years to afford to have.

My mind was racing to find a solution. "Should I just leave you here to enjoy yourself while I drive to San Jose to get the fucking purse and come back to pick you up?" I pathetically offered.

"No. The point of coming here was to enjoy the day with you, so if you stay or go it doesn't matter because it's already ruined. Just give me some fucking space and stop whimpering." He stormed out of the parking garage with me in tow. He just kept walking. He knew I had to follow. I had no money.

Nothing. I was helpless and I deserved to suffer for leaving my fucking purse in the fucking closet because of the fucking cat. I was crying and he told me to shut up. He just wanted me to shut the fuck up. He didn't want to hear me cry. He didn't want to hear a peep. Just leave him alone. (But follow him.)

"Should we just separate and meet somewhere in a few hours?" I offered, still desperate to find a viable solution.

No, he didn't want to discuss a thing. I had to follow him because what else could I do? What were my plans? What was I going to do if I didn't have his money to feed me and get my fucking car out of the garage?

I thought, *Why can't he just pay for everything just for today and not give a shit and not ruin the end of our vacation*? I was not and never would be worried that I'd lost my wallet, especially in a major city in the United States. Someone could wire me money. I could go to an American Express office. I'd be resourceful. I tried to apologize, but at the same time was furious that he was so furious over something so small, which I'm sure had shone right through my apology.

We walked around the city, him leading and screaming, me crying and following him like a dog trying to stop crying because he told me I shouldn't have the nerve to mortify him on the street when I was the one who caused all of this drama. He finally walked us back to the garage. I drove to the exit, and he paid to get the car out of the garage. And he paid for the gas at the gas station. It was a torture-filled drive of complete silence for hours and hours. And then, finally, John asked me a question.

"Where is it that you planned for us to stay the night?" he tried to calmly ask.

"Well, I actually didn't have a plan," I admitted.

"I thought you said you knew of a place," he fumed.

"I said I was sure we'd find a place in Santa Barbara. Why don't we just forget it and go home, it's only another two hours."

"Didn't we already plan to stay in Santa Barbara?" he wanted to know. "Why would we have to change our plans just because you are so irresponsible? Our entire trip shouldn't have to be ruined because of you. If it's so easy to find a place in Santa Barbara, then find one."

It seemed he couldn't wait for me to fuck up again. We weren't having a remotely good time, so I couldn't understand why he wanted to stick to the plan. He kept asking where I thought we were going to stay as if the question hadn't been asked and answered. *Jesus fucking Christ, get the fuck off my back*, I didn't have the nerve to say because he'd started to convince me that I actually had fucked him over as hard as he thought I had.

We found the worst, cheesiest, trying-to-be-fancy place and checked in. John thought that because here he was paying so much for such a nice hotel that I had better shape up and act like I was enjoying it. I shouldn't have the nerve to not like anything when he had to pay for everything because I didn't have my purse. *Who had John become? What was happening?*

The room had two doubles. We slept separately and drove home the next morning in an exhausted silence that was palpably simmering with rage. Hours later, we were supposed to be at his thirty-third birthday dinner with a small group of his closest friends. I was so disturbed by the weekend and disgusted with John that the last thing I wanted to do was celebrate him. But he was even more furious when he learned I didn't want to go. I had to fuck up the weekend *and* his birthday? If I felt that way, fine, because the last thing he wanted was to have to worry about me not acting right in front of his friends. And I couldn't believe that he cared more about his friends than he did about me and our relationship.

I decided that I didn't want to not be there, making his birthday more of a drama with all of his friends asking where I was. So I went and I went feeling beaten. I could barely act okay but didn't want to act sour because that would piss him off. And I gave him a very nice present that I had already bought, six pairs of great socks—some cashmere, some patterned, some plain—and a dark brown belt to match the dark brown shoes I had already bought him for our first anniversary. And he was happy with the gifts and we were miserable with each other.

thirty

my weekly report

As ashamed as I was by the way I'd let myself be treated and the way that the guy who supposedly loved me saw fit to treat me, I had no choice but to tell DLB everything. After she carefully listened to me struggle through my rendition, she told me something I was shocked to hear. DLB said John's behavior was abusive.

DLB explained that more often than not, abusive people are the last people one might suspect are abusive because they are so loving and generous and kind to everyone at work or at the grocery store or wherever. But it is that very person who goes home and beats the shit out of his wife or his children. Abusers could easily blame the ones they abused because they were able to prove to themselves that they were really nice people, as evidenced by the world's response to their charm. As she spoke I thought of how much John was universally loved by everyone at work, from the hair and makeup people down to the security guards. They couldn't imagine a nicer guy. Of course John wasn't remotely beating the shit out of me, but he was starting to be verbally abusive . . . I couldn't believe the word "abusive" was coming up in my therapy session. Oh shit. Could it be true? Could I, a strong, educated, confident woman, be in an abusive relationship? How and when did that happen? Had it happened? Had I let it?

Between the verbal abuse and our sexless sex life, DLB strongly recommended we go to couples therapy. However, she explained that she could not be our couples therapist because, as my therapist, she might not appear impartial to John. "Would you like some recommendations?" she asked.

Shaking, I nodded my head.

On the way out I gave her John's urologist's report. The doctor said Propecia was not to blame. She wasn't surprised.

thirty-one

what will honey and julius think?

Because things were obviously going so well between John and me, we decided to move in together. Unfortunately for us, we were more concerned about what my grandparents would think about it than we were about what we thought. We didn't take the time to discuss the ramifications of this big step. Instead, it seemed our decision was born more out of convenience than anything else.

Despite not being a Jew and despite working in a totally unreliable profession, John had quickly become the star of the family. No one could help themselves. Everybody loved John. Grandmother Honey especially. She craved his attention, loved improvising with him, and lived for sitting next to him in the backseat of her and Grandpa's car, where she'd hold his hand for the length of the ride. Even Grandpa liked John and was happy there was finally someone with whom he could talk sports, whom he could make listen to his latest incomprehensible investment scheme.

And I'm sure it didn't hurt that John was experiencing some financial success. My grandparents couldn't help themselves, they just had to know how much an actor on TV made—specifically an actor who was dating their granddaughter. So one day while I was chauffeuring them in their car, Grandmother took the opportunity to inquire.

"What kind of remuneration does John receive for acting on his show?" Grandmother asked as nonchalantly as she could, as if her word choice didn't give away that she'd been thinking of the most delicate way to ask the question.

Like the time when Grandmother asked me why I never had a date, this was another rare instance when Grandpa didn't yell at Grandmother to be quiet. While I was driving.

I was proud to have the opportunity to calmly answer, "Fifteen thousand dollars a week." I looked forward to what they were going to say to that!

"You mean fifteen hundred, don't you?" my perked-up grandpa asked, as if he thought nothing of talking while the car was moving.

"No, fifteen thousand. Actually, he makes fifteen thousand five hundred to be exact."

They were in awe. They couldn't come up with anything to say. I wouldn't say that his salary made them love him even more, but it certainly made them more proud to tell their doctors, dentists, lawyers, and bank tellers that their granddaughter's boyfriend was on a TV show. Had they seen it?

And while they couldn't have been happier with John and me, it seemed they certainly could have been a hell of a lot happier with my cousin Marney and her now-fiancé Noah. My grandparents told John and me what they would never have told Marney and Noah directly. Instead, as usual, they chose to show their disapproval without a word of explanation, leaving Marney and Noah to wonder what they'd done to upset them. I was used to/only knew this form of communication, whereas John couldn't believe the way my family attempted to communicate and control one another.

Grandmother and Grandpa did not approve of Marney and Noah's wedding plans. They thought a big wedding was a total waste of money. I was surprised to hear it, as I considered my grandparents the king and queen of party-throwing. As a child, I loved to look at all of the glamorous photos of them in their heyday. I marveled at Grandmother's glamorous gowns, her jewels, her furs, her poodle's furs, Grandpa's dapper white dinner jackets,

In their heyday, my grandparents were the king and queen of party-giving. I couldn't believe that they thought Marney and Noah should be denied a wedding just because they were living together.

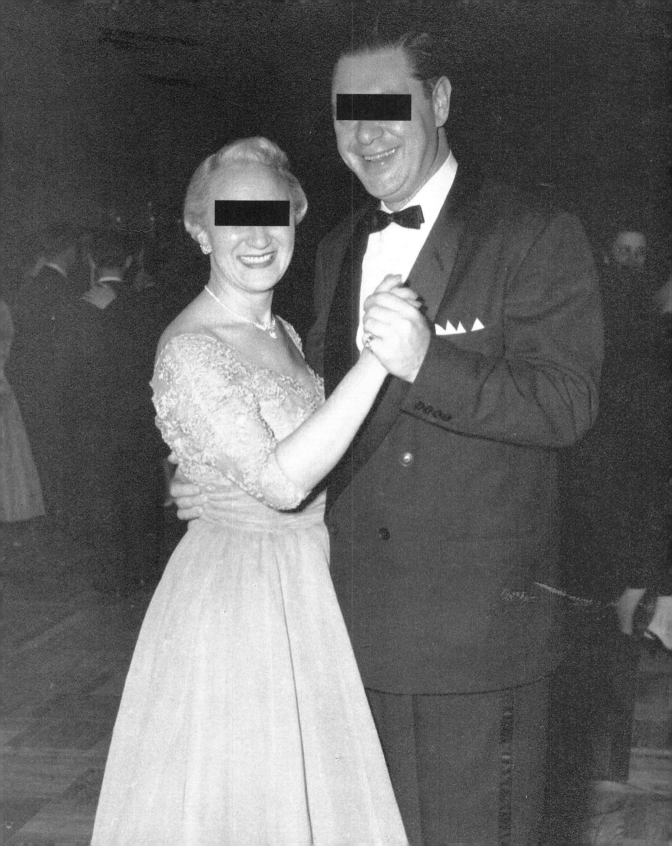

his tuxes, the bands. I ate up the formality of their very social social life. My mother's wedding was exquisite. Even my grandparents' recent sixtieth anniversary party was rather lavish. What were they talking about? Weren't they excited that finally there was something to celebrate? Finally one of their three almost-past-marrying-age (from their point of view) granddaughters was getting married. Isn't this what they'd wanted for soooooo long? Isn't this the occasion they thought they'd be dead for?

Instead, Grandmother wondered aloud to us, "What's there to celebrate? Marney and Noah have already been living together for two years. Why bother with an expensive wedding?"

"They should take the twenty-five K we're giving them as a wedding gift and do something useful with it. Not just blow it on some dinner and dancing," Grandpa chimed in.

The way my grandparents decided to communicate their disapproval was to refuse to walk down the aisle at their wedding and pretend that the reason was because Grandpa didn't have a tuxedo. Meanwhile, by telling John and me the truth of the matter, they were more than likely subconsciously counting on me to convey (to another family member, who would tell another family member, who would tell Marney) what they really meant when they called to tell Marney and Noah that they wouldn't be walking down the aisle. Indirect communication was my family's trademark.

Still unable to extricate myself from the communication web—despite the progress I'd made with the Notorious DLB—I called my mom with my outrage at her parents' behavior. Why were they doing this to Marney and Noah, who had so many other problems to deal with?

Cut to my dad in Grandpa's closet finding his tuxes. Cut to my dad chauffeuring Grandpa to the tailor. Cut to Grandmother calling Marney on Grandpa's behalf with their *new* reason for not walking down the aisle. Grandpa's back was too crooked now and he didn't want people to have the opportunity to focus on his embarrassing condition—as if people expected eighty-seven-year-old men to stand perfectly straight.

Apparently, my grandparents didn't care that Marney and Noah were being pulled in so many directions by a slew of parents, stepparents, ex-stepparents, and the like during what was supposed to be a time of joy. They had a statement to make about how Noah and Marney had handled their relationship. After they felt like they'd caused enough commotion—just hours before the nuptials were to begin—they changed their mind and decided to walk down the god-damned aisle. Filled with pride, joy, and gallons of amnesia, they walked down the aisle, loving every second of it. They thought it was an exquisite affair.

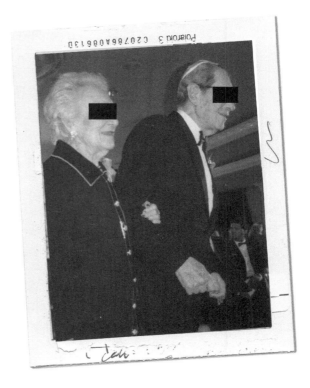

John observed these shenanigans, incredulous. In order to avoid any veiled protests at our not-impending nuptials, John wanted to confront my grandparents head-on about any misgivings they might have about us moving in together. Comfortable in my perfect-granddaughter role, I, of course, was afraid to tell them anything. They seemed pretty well set in their ways.

Of course, my grandparents did end up walking down the aisle at Marney and Noah's wedding. They never wouldn't have. They just had something to say and couldn't think of any other way of saying it.

John suggested I ask my mother, their daughter, for advice—not realizing that I didn't feel comfortable talking to my mother about such things. The last conversation I wanted to have with my mother was about how serious my relationship with John was or wasn't. When she was next over at my place, I literally forced myself to blurt out that John was moving in. And then before I lost my chutzpah, I was quick to ask what she thought I should say to her sure-to-be-disapproving parents.

"I won't say anything to them," she promised, by way of advice.

Her response was to help me keep a secret that I didn't want to keep! I guess she, too, was comfortable in her perfect-daughter role. She probably figured that they were too old to change their thinking, so why upset them? I thought it must really be a problem if my mom was advocating lying/truth withholding.

"Not to worry," John said, "I have a plan. We have to invite your grandparents out for dinner and tell them directly. Respectfully acknowledging their disapproval is the only way."

"Being direct is your family's Achilles' heel," John explained. "When you tell them what they don't want to hear directly to their face with love and respect, they crumble." He was such a stand-up guy. I was so lucky and so nervous. He was nervous, too, but more titillated by the challenge than anything. My grandparents were delighted with the invitation. For days before the big night, John paced our apartment practicing his speech.

The big night came, and while John was nervous driving over in the car, I was a wreck. I wanted nothing more than for the night to have already played itself out and for us to be on our way home. We met my grandparents at a Beverly Hills nouveau Asian restaurant, kissed, hugged, and sat down. The waitress soon asked us if she could bring us drinks, to which Grandmother asked, "Are you also an actress? It seems that every waiter in this city is one."

"Yes, I am, ma'am," she politely responded.

"Well, so is John here. As a matter of fact, he's on a TV show! We hope it lasts." *This is going to be fun*, I thought, trying to apologize to the poor waitress with my eyes.

John waited until the drinks and appetizers came before he began—he didn't want any interruptions. *Let this night end, let me be at home in bed watching TV, reflecting back on what has already taken place instead of anticipating it*, I begged the god of time. The appetizers came. *Here we go* . . . I steeled myself.

John started rather formally, "Mr. and Mrs. K., thank you for accepting our invitation to join us for dinner this evening. As you know, Jennifer and I have something very important that we want to talk to you about." They probably started hearing wedding bells. "I'm sure that you will have many questions. I ask only that you hear me out and save your questions until I am finished, at which time Jennifer and I will be happy to answer them the best we can." He was so impressive—a real man.

"We want you to know, and we wanted to tell you in person, that Jennifer and I have decided to live together. This is not a decision that we take lightly. In this day and age, when divorce is so common, most couples live together first to see if they are compatible. My parents divorced and I do not want to make the same mistake. Our situation is hard—what with me living in Venice and Jennifer in West Hollywood. In traffic, it can take an hour from home to home! I had thought about simply moving into Jennifer's neighborhood, as I could certainly afford it, but I thought that it would be a waste of money, seeing that we spend so much time together." He kept reiterating how we don't take this step in our relationship lightly. He made sure they understood that we didn't confuse living together with marriage. "As a matter of fact," he slipped in, "we plan on going to the *mikvah* before we get married—should we get married—to symbolize the significant change in our lives from living together to marriage."

When he was good and finished, John asked them if they had any questions. All the appetizers were gone, which didn't stop Grandpa and me from continuing to wipe the sauce on the plate with whatever scrap of food we managed to hold on to. After a nine-months-long pregnant pause, Grandpa said, "That all sounds well and good, but it can't go on forever. You should make a decision by my eighty-eighth birthday." The way he saw it, we had less than a year to get on with things.

Then Grandmother had a question. "You mentioned a *mikvah*"—the Jewish ritual bath. "As I understand it, that is only for Orthodox women."

She played right into his hands. "Well, Honey, yes, that is true. Orthodox women do go to the *mikvah* monthly, actually. But today, in both the Conservative and Reform practices, many brides and grooms go to the *mikvah* before their wedding to demark the new and important stage in their life. Jennifer and I have met with a rabbi and have talked about this," John explained—not revealing that we were taking the very course that she was dying to have him take. Very impressed, if not dumbfounded, Grandmother nodded her head. The food came. John had triumphed. My hero. Facing things head-on. I never could have done it. They loved him even more. There was no question, they would be walking down the aisle at our wedding without some bullshit protest. They'd have bells on. Would I?

thirty-two

couples therapy

John's therapist, Robert, had seconded the Notorious DLB's couples-therapy recommend-ation. However, Robert didn't feel it was as imper-ative that we see a third, impartial couples therapist. John told me that he and Robert had discussed us seeing Robert because that way his insurance would cover the visits. Just what DLB had warned me against! *Why did this have to be so difficult*?

While I was annoyed that someone making as much money a week as John was felt he needed to skimp on something as obviously important as couples therapy, I knew that he was scared—very scared. He was starting to see the handwriting on the wall. He didn't think he'd be asked back to the show next season—if there was going to be another season. He already knew they were firing the father, and given the fact that he rarely got anything to do, he didn't think it looked good for him. And even though the show was stupid and he was miserable doing nothing on it, he still wanted to be asked back. Everyone wants to be wanted and who wouldn't want another $350,000? And who wants to face the embarrassment of being fired? And worse yet, who wants to go from having something going on to nothing? So even though he was raking it in, John was busy preparing for the worst, busy panicking about his future, busy feeling like a failure, busy being nervous about what people would think of his failure, busy not wanting to waste any money on couples therapy when there was a viable alternative. Robert was a good therapist, he assured me.

I couldn't understand why if DLB was so worried about not appearing impartial, Robert wasn't. I could only guess that perhaps Robert reasoned that in light of John's financial fears, seeing him was better than us going elsewhere only to have John resent the expense. Nonetheless, I had to get an okay from DLB.

"It's better than nothing," she said, adding, "You can always go see someone else if it doesn't work out."

Oh gosh, it was taking so long to just get started. John had to first ask Robert, then report to me, then I had to ask DLB and report to John, who then had to make an appointment with Robert. And then we had to see Robert long enough to judge if his being John's therapist would or would not impede our progress. When was the beginning of the end of our fighting and fucked-up sex life going to begin? When was John going to swoon over me again like I continued to swoon over him in between our fights? (I did find it remarkable how quickly I'd forgive him and find myself aching for his love and his gorgeous ass.)

John and Robert finally set an appointment. We'd go the Friday after we came back from our mini-trip to the desert, where I was hoping he'd want to kiss me and love me and screw me even though we'd yet to set a foot into couples therapy. And John was hoping, too. He was hoping the quiet and the stars and the desert would jump-start his libido. He couldn't believe the Propecia wasn't to blame.

thirty-three
motherfucking desert

I had made reservations at the 29 Palms Inn—an inexpensive, low-key place just outside the Joshua Tree National Park. How lucky we were that John had a job that gave him every fourth week off.

Our first day, we went on a mind-blowing hike. For a while everything looked like I had expected—big rocks and cacti everywhere. But then when we went farther and farther and higher and higher, we turned our heads in a different direction, and suddenly, the landscape was prehistoric, very *Land of the Lost*. We climbed around some more, jumped from rock to rock, and sang.

The trip was going great except that I was in a perpetual state of monitoring how much John was or was not being affectionate. *Why isn't he putting his arm around me? Is he going to make out with me and make me feel like he was so happy to have the time to love me the way I should be loved or not? Is he going to finally fuck me tonight?* Before I had a chance to find out, based on the evidence I'd been gathering all afternoon, I had already worked myself up into a he-doesn't-love-me frenzy before dinner and started to cry.

John was surprisingly sympathetic. He put his arm around me and asked what was wrong. I whimpered something about wanting love and he did his best to reassure me that he did love me, very much. At the inn restaurant,

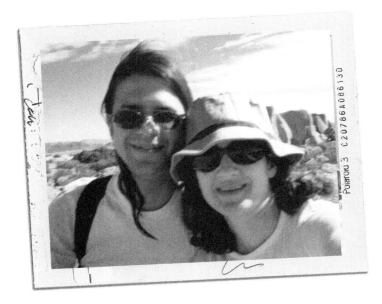

Happy hikers, we had no idea that as soon as the sun set we'd be outraged by each other, one degree away from breaking up.

John did his best to keep the conversation going and it seemed that I pulled out of my despair enough to talk without weeping.

Then we went back to our room and got in bed and watched TV. We lay there watching and watching. *When was something going to happen?* I wondered. All I could think about was that he wasn't touching me or at least not in the making-a-pass way that I wanted/expected him to and that he knew I wanted him to. If he did love me like he said he did, and if he was so looking forward to this vacation like he said he was, then what was the problem? Seeing that it had worked for me earlier in the evening, I started to cry.

Well, it was just more than he could take—my constant neediness was too much. Why couldn't he just relax after the constant nonstop stress of his job? Why couldn't I just let things happen? Why was I so controlling? Why couldn't we just have a great hike, a romantic walk under the stars, a nice dinner, and get in bed and watch a concert on TV?

Within seconds I was off and running. I'd had it with not being loved the way I was dying to be loved and being made to feel like there was something wrong with me for wanting it. I was a young woman who needed to be fucked.

John was furious at me for screaming. The neighbors could hear! The more he wanted me to quiet down, the louder I got. Fuck him for caring more about the neighbors' needs than mine! Fifteen minutes of our worst-fight-ever later, I threatened to just leave him there by himself. He could find his own way back to Los Angeles. I didn't need this shit. I got in my car and skidded out of there.

After driving around the little desert ghost town for about a half hour in the middle of the night, I came back. And even though my tears had subsided, my stomach hurt with the pain of knowing I was in a relationship I shouldn't be in. We somehow managed to sleep in the same bed together but the next morning we erupted again and I cried—on and off hysterically—almost the entire two-and-a-half-hour ride home. And with each tear I shed, he got madder and madder and felt more and more trapped. What had he done to deserve this shit? Why did I insist on ruining all of our trips? Did I think this was the way to get him to want to love me the way I wanted to be loved?

I dropped John off at my apartment that I was regretting was now our apartment and went to Jason's for a sleepover. By now Jason was used to me coming over. I was too worn-out to go into anything. I'd had it. Didn't I deserve to be loved and properly fucked? I hated John. And I hated our relationship.

thirty-four

motherfucking white knuckles

I couldn't wait the two days until our appointment with Robert, I had to talk to someone right away—so I called my first-kiss friend Derek on my cell. Two minutes in I had to pull my car over because I was crying too hard to drive—let alone speak. Between jags, I told him that John and I were fighting all the time. That I felt misunderstood. That he did. That John was miserable on his stupid TV show. That John was playing Nintendo all the time and didn't like to be disturbed. That he gave the cat more attention than he did me. That we weren't having sex—at all. What was I doing with someone like that?

Derek, a recovering alcoholic with ten years of sobriety who knew John back when he woke up on people's lawns after a heavy night of drinking, had a single question that he already knew the answer to: "Is John working or has John worked the steps?"

"I don't know," I whimpered. "He goes to an AA meeting in Venice every Sunday."

"Yes, but does he work the steps? Does he have a sponsor?"

"I don't know," I whimpered again, realizing I'd never given it any thought.

"How long has he been sober now?" he asked.

"Maybe two years, maybe less," I guessed.

"Sounds to me like he's white-knuckling it."

"What does that mean?"

"It means that even though you aren't drinking, you aren't sober. We call them dry drunks—someone who thinks that by simply not putting alcohol in your system, you are cured—as if sobriety only has to do with willpower. If you have stopped drinking but you haven't worked the steps that are designed to help alcoholics deal with the shit that drove them to drink in the first place, then you have no way to work through your feelings and on top of that you aren't drinking to self-medicate, so you have no outlet for your pain at all. Dry drunks actually feel worse than active drunks. And it would make total sense that he is having problems with sex and intimacy. Most alcoholics do until they've worked the steps."

What is wrong with me? I thought. *How could I just have ignored the fact that John is an alcoholic? Or not so much ignored it but not given any thought to it?* I was shocked at my stupidity. But it made sense and it gave me hope. John could work the steps to make our life better. He wasn't not attracted to me or not in love with me, he was a dry drunk. What a relief. Fuck.

Even though I knew John went to meetings, I never stopped for a second to think what he got out of them. I didn't even think to inquire about the twelve steps of AA's twelve-step program. I didn't know there was a difference between just attending meetings and "working the program." All I knew was that when we started dating he had been sober for over a year and that he looked a million times better than he did when I first saw him perform years earlier. He'd put some weight on his rail-thin body. His skin had cleared up. He'd quit his two-to-three-pack-a-day smoking habit. He seemed totally recovered to me. I had just naively thought, *Well, great. That's over with.* I knew he was sober and in therapy, therefore datable. I thought I was avoiding my tracks with him, but was I?

Derek advised me, as someone in a relationship with an alcoholic—recovering or otherwise—to go to Al-Anon meetings. "Your behavior is codependent, which you probably don't realize. While it's true John is behaving like an asshole, the way you respond does nothing to help. And you have to learn how to live with a recovering alcoholic. You should go today if you can." he implored, "I know you'll find some relief."

Fuck! I can't believe I have to go to fucking Al-Anon meetings when I'm not the one with a problem, I thought, as if it wasn't my problem that I was attracted to someone with such a serious problem. I was afraid. I didn't want to have to call Information and find the number for Al-Anon. I didn't want to have to call for a schedule and then choose a meeting and then go and introduce myself like I'd seen in the movies. I didn't want to have to say, "Hi, my name is Jennifer, and I'm a newcomer." I didn't want to have to hear everyone say back, "Hello, Jennifer." I didn't want to then feel nervous about sharing. But I had to. I was in love with an alcoholic, a dry drunk, a guy with ten motherfucking white knuckles, and there *was* something I could do about it. I was devastated by my predicament.

I had to talk to John right away. Anytime I had a serious realization of some kind, I had to share it with him. I was sure he was getting sick of my diagnoses: it's your job, the rabbi, Propecia, alcoholism that's ruining our lives. I managed to tell him that I thought he was white-knuckling it and I knew that there was nothing I could do to make him work the steps but I could go to Al-Anon meetings, which I had every intention of doing. I made myself tell him that so I would be forced to live up to my side of the bargain.

Without acknowledging the dry-drunk concept I'd put forth, he simply said he thought Al-Anon was a great idea. He was glad to see me taking some responsibility, as opposed to blaming him all the time. That was fine with me because at least soon we'd be going to couples therapy with his therapist, so I'd have a chance to get Robert to realize John was white-knuckling it and then he could take it from there. Meanwhile, I could talk a good game, but I didn't go online to find out when and where meetings were. I didn't do dick.

thirty-five
motherfucking couples therapy

On our long drive in Friday traffic to John's therapist Robert's totally inconvenient office (way out past Marina del Rey), I wondered what he was going to be like and what he'd think of me. John liked Robert. He felt he really cared about him and liked how he talked about living authentically, about becoming an authentic person.

After waiting in Robert's waiting room fifteen minutes past the time of our appointment, I—already eager to find something wrong with him because I thought we should be seeing an impartial therapist—became suspicious of his professionalism. DLB would never start a session late! Finally a man and his little girl walked out followed by a friendly-faced, big-bellied older man who said hello and how nice it was to meet me.

"Come on in. John has told me so many wonderful things about you," Robert warmly said. I was sure he had heard some not so wonderful things about me, too. "John told me about the night that you were really there for him at his show. You know, your support really meant a lot to him."

Robert was talking about John's big moment on the sitcom. Junior was going to break his vow of silence to save his sister, the Beautiful Blonde, from her lying, deceitful, smarmy ex—the father of her child—who had weaseled his way back into her heart. As usual, John got the script at the beginning of the week and found out how he'd be breaking his vow of silence:

```
                        JUNIOR:
     He's telling the truth. I saw him in the bushes when I
     was driving home from the dry cleaners.
```

The audience would at once be shocked that Junior was speaking and relieved that the Beautiful Blonde wasn't going back to the father-of-her-child asshole when she could find true happiness with the Latin Lover.

They had rehearsed all week and the script went through all of its changes, but Junior's two lines never changed. Then, on the day they were going to film the show at 4:30 P.M., about an hour before they were going to start, the writers didn't change John's lines but instead added a monologue. They wanted to show how ironic/funny it was that Junior—truly a genius who had an extensive vocabulary—had chosen not to speak for all of these years. To illustrate this, they strung together a bunch of big fancy words into a complex paragraph that ultimately meant nothing. It was as dumb as this:

```
                        JUNIOR:
     And by the way I find it strange that the conflated
     infrastructure  of  the  metaphysical  atmospheric
     assumptions, based on a bifurcated interpretation of a
     Socratic, and must I mention, plagiarized theory, are
     totally  antithetical  when  considering  all  of  the
     previously proven Hegelian theorems in the context of the
     various trajectories.
```

After nine episodes of pointing and juggling and raising his eyebrows, John had his big moment and he couldn't for the life of him remember his convoluted poor-excuse-for-lines. There was too little time, too much pressure, and too many words no one ever used, particularly in the order they were written. He was an absolute wreck sitting in his trailer in full makeup and costume trying desperately to remember his monologue. I had showed up soon after he'd received the rewrite and had never seen anything like it. John was sweating, he was on the verge of tears, he was panicked but trying not to overwhelm himself because he had to get these lines. He felt the weight of the world on his shoulders. He had to show his bosses, fellow actors, and crew of two hundred that he was an actor who *could* memorize lines and give a good reading—something he hadn't had to do for the small fortune he'd already been paid. His job, his pride, his self-esteem, his career depended on flawlessly delivering these stupid fucking lines. He had until the last scene of the night to get them down. The next six hours were among the most painful of his life, right up there with spending the night in jail tripping on acid knowing he was facing five years in prison. (By the grace of God, both felonies and misdemeanors were later dropped due to faulty paperwork.)

On my way over to Warner Brothers, I was once again worked up, having come from therapy with the Notorious DLB. I had every intention of finding a time suitable to John when we could discuss some more of the things I wasn't going to take from him anymore. But my anger turned to empathy the moment I saw this poor sweet scared guy whom I really did love so much, whom I would do anything to help. My poor baby. I did what I could. I ran the lines with him over and over and over and over and over again and desperately tried to think of ways for him to remember what phrase was next. I was furious at the fucking writers. *Why couldn't they have come up with anything sooner and anything better*? *Don't they realize what they're doing*? *How can they think someone could memorize all of this shit in five fucking minutes*? I was like a lion defending her pup.

Periodically John had to go shoot a scene. He'd put on his smile, enter the soundstage, dance with the cast, and tell jokes in between takes. Then he'd come back to me totally panicked. The pressure was too high and his confidence in his ability to memorize too low. He was psyching himself out.

He was an improviser, not a memorizer. He started to cry. I told him that he could do it and that it would be okay. We continued to run the lines again and again. Never once did he get them right.

Finally, six hours later, the fucking scene came. The Beautiful Blonde said her line, the smarmy father of her child said his, the Latin Lover said his, back to the BB, and then Junior started to say his as the studio audience gasped that Junior was actually talking and then Junior launched into his monologue and stopped. Fuck.

"Lines," he called. He needed the script supervisor to review his lines with him while the audience, crew, cast, and producers waited. I couldn't fucking take it. I couldn't imagine how he was going to do it. John nodded; he was ready to go.

"Quiet on the set," yelled the assistant director.

"We've got speed," followed the cameraman.

"Action," called the director.

Again, it went from the BB to the father of her child to the LL to the BB as my heart pounded harder and harder.

Then it was John's turn.

```
                    JUNIOR:
And by the way I find it strange that the
conflated infrastructure of the atmospheric
interpretations bifurcated just saying
Socratic ideas involved things and other
interpretations
```

"Cut," yelled the director after it became clear that John was just going for it despite the fact that he didn't remember the actual lines.

Holy shit, my poor Angelhead, I thought, my heart racing, not knowing how this evening would ever end.

The producers and writers all huddled together and then a miracle happened: they decided to cut the monologue altogether. All he had to say was his original two lines. All of that heartache for NOTHING.

Robert reiterated how much my support had meant to John. I said that I was glad I could be there for him, that I wished I could have done more.

Robert and his office were the exact opposite of DLB's scene. DLB was beautiful—tall, thin, and well dressed. Her pants hung perfectly, her hair was tastefully highlighted, and her makeup was meticulously applied so that you didn't notice she was wearing any. Her office was chic and serene with a built-in sectional and glass coffee table. Robert's scene, however, was more Formica and Office Depot. Robert had a tight big belly that prevented his blazer button from closing. I couldn't help thinking that I wanted a couples therapist who was a great role model, meaning that he could balance things in his life like not eating too much and exercising. After the small talk, it was time to talk about why we were there.

I started to recount the San Francisco purse disaster but didn't get very far. I'd start to say something and John would interrupt and refute it. He'd try to explain and downplay his behavior and I'd interrupt to explain to Robert that in fact it was as bad as I was saying it was. As we continued to interrupt and defend, interrupt and defend, exasperation and anger filled up our bodies and infiltrated our voice boxes. We were both fuming that the other didn't see how obviously wrong s/he had been. Our tones were ugly and our language even uglier.

Rather quickly and totally unfortunately, Robert took my side. He even used the A-word. And John flipped the fuck out.

"I was not and have never been abusive. Jennifer's totally exaggerating. I love Jennifer. I'd never hit her. Ever!" John angrily said.

"John, I never said that you hit Jennifer. What I meant is that I would classify the way you treated Jennifer in San Francisco as verbally abusive," Robert calmly explained.

I was at once relieved and scared that Robert was saying to John what DLB had said to me. I never would have had the nerve to even mention it to

John myself. And this was why. I was afraid of John going ballistic—which was precisely why we were there. Well, that and the fact that we didn't have sex anymore. I naively thought the two were unrelated.

John couldn't believe that *his* therapist was taking *my* side. Robert didn't even know me, let alone know the whole story. How did this turn into a John-is-an-abusive-guy-and-is-totally-in-the-wrong couples-therapy session? John figured Robert would never blame me—someone he barely knew—having just met me, right off the bat like that. This wasn't fair. Exclamation mark times thirty million.

The Notorious DLB was right! And I had seen this coming, just ten minutes into the session. Why couldn't Robert see that everything he was saying made John feel that he was taking my side? As we continued, I was becoming increasingly afraid of what Robert was going to say next because I knew it was going to make John feel more and more ganged up on—even though Robert was so calm and gentle when he spoke. Didn't Robert realize that I had to sleep with John that night? John fumed for the rest of the session but didn't tell Robert how betrayed by him he felt. The ride home was excruciating. John hated me and his therapist and I hated John, his stupid therapist for being so stupid, and DLB for letting me go in the first place.

But we dutifully returned for yet another session of John feeling betrayed during which Robert did manage to convey some useful ideas. Robert explained that if we weren't so busy interrupting each other, if we weren't so busy thinking of how what the other person said wasn't true, we had a better chance of hearing what our partner was really saying. To our rescue was "I" messages. Robert asked us to review the handout.

"I" Messages

The point is to get your "here-and-now" needs met as often as possible. If you attack or blame the other person, he will not be able to meet your needs, as he will spend his energy defending himself.

I didn't know what a "here-and-now" need was. But I understood the "defending himself" part. I was always telling John why his feelings about something I had done were wrong due to his misunderstanding of what I had actually done and why I had done it. He wouldn't feel the way he was feeling if he only knew the truth.

> Your task is to find out what's really going on in your inner world and describe this to the other person.

Inner world? I was lost already.

1. Neutral Description of the Situation. No blame, no solutions. (Don't tell the other person how to meet your needs.)

2. Your Feelings. Reveal without blaming the other person for your feelings. They may be a product of your own unfinished business or your own unique personality. Nevertheless, those feelings are you at the moment and are important and valuable information for you and your partner to know and respect. (If you are receiving an "I" message, be careful about "hooking in" and taking responsibility for your partner's heavy feelings. Instead, hear his feelings and decide whether you will meet his needs or not and how you want to do it.)

Ahh, that I understood. I was certainly prone to "hooking in." I always felt bad when John felt bad, as if it was my fault. I couldn't ever be calm if he was upset. I never felt I had an option about whether or not I should meet his needs, as my instinct was to just meet his needs to make him feel better.

And then the handout went on to tell what common errors were, what good examples of "I" messages were, and what good examples of follow-ups to "I" messages were. The handout said that anger is often a secondary feeling, a response to deeper and more specific feelings like fear, hurt, embarrassment, jealousy, and disappointment. That sharing these feelings instead of anger will have a greater impact. This one sheet was one of a dozen or so sheets Robert gave us.

There was the "Baker's Dirty Dozen Blocks to Communication" that cleverly listed the things a couple should *not* do if they want to truly communicate with each other.

1. Directing, commanding: You must . . .
2. Warning, threatening: You had better . . .
3. Advising, providing solutions: Why don't you . . .
4. Judging negatively, blaming: It's your fault that . . .

There were eight more and I was guilty of a lot them—primarily number three! Flipping through the stack of handouts, I started to become overwhelmed. There was Communication Strategies Guaranteed to Create Conflict in Marriage; the Eight Hot Potatoes of Marriage; "Fair Fighting" Guidelines; Paraphrase—A Basic Communication Skill; Examples of Dysfunctional Communication Patterns; Individual and Interpersonal Style; Enhancing Companionship in Marriage; Maintaining Personal Boundaries in Relationships; Why People Fear Closeness; the Ten Commandments of Communication; and finally, Negotiating Conflicts. *Holy shit!* I thought. *I didn't know about any of this stuff! And how am I even supposed to remember any of it when we're in the middle of a fight?*

We took our packet home, read through it, were sufficiently overwhelmed by the work we had to do, grabbed a manila file that I labeled RELATIONSHIP, dropped the sheets in the file, dropped the file in the drawer, and closed it.

Finally, in one of his individual sessions, John mustered the nerve to tell Robert how betrayed by him he felt when he took what John perceived as my side. Fortunately, they both determined that seeing Robert for couples therapy wasn't such a great idea after all. John could have his ther-

apist back and I could finally call the referrals the Notorious DLB had origi-
nally given me. Maybe now we could realistically get on our way to becoming happy people who knew how to communicate and liked to screw.

Meanwhile, I took some of Robert's sheets out of the file drawer and put
them on my bedside table to review each night before I went to sleep. And
even though I was annoyed that Robert and John had not heeded DLB's
warning regarding not using a neutral couples therapist, I thought it was
helpful that Robert had had a chance to see a more out-of-control side of
John that surely he never would've seen without me there to provoke it.
Now I was confident that Robert would clearly see that John was a white-
knuckling-it alcoholic and would be attending to John's verbal "A"-ness. I
felt like I'd led my horse to water.

thirty-six

harville

The following week's show night at Warner Brothers Soundstage 8, John's attorney, Craig, came to check out the scene. John was back and forth between his trailer and the soundstage, but I stayed in his trailer most of the night hosting Craig and my friend Julie. The conversation quickly veered toward relationships, breakups, and therapy. Craig started to talk about this amazing weekend program he had attended with his former girlfriend. "Even though it obviously didn't work for us as we are no longer together, the weekend was incredibly valuable—I can't recommend it highly enough. It was based on the work of psychologist Harville Hendrix, author of this book *Getting the Love You Want*. Have you heard of him?"

"No," I said, totally interested in every word that was coming out of his mouth. Images of John and me staring nervously at each other in a room full of other couples flashed in my head. I wanted to get the love I wanted.

So Craig launched into his version of Harville's theory of love and relationships, which was a lot easier for me to digest than Robert's five hundred how-to-respectfully/efficiently-communicate sheets.

"We are the result of our upbringing, of the way our parents did or didn't love us, did or didn't listen to us, were or were not affectionate with us, and perhaps most importantly the way our parents did or didn't love each other. Inevitably, we are people with issues, problems, whatever . . . we aren't whole. Let's say . . ." Craig continued. "For the sake of illustration, let's say that those problems have manifested themselves physically. Okay, so let's say my problem is that I have only one right arm and one right leg because my other arm and leg were not encouraged to grow. But I get by. Then one day I find a woman whom I find attractive. It turns out her problems perfectly complement mine—what with her one left arm and one left leg. Together, we feel whole. Now, with our two arms and legs, we can walk around the world with ease. Life is perfect, we are happy, we are deliriously happy . . . we have fallen in love."

He had my attention.

"But after a while, I might want to walk in a different direction than this new love of my life. I might want to walk faster or slower, or I might want to walk to the bar when she wants to walk home and get in bed and watch TV. And I start to become annoyed with this new love of my life when she doesn't want to do what I want to do when I want to do it. I am so surprised. What happened? We'd been walking together so beautifully, so perfectly, for so long, some six months, maybe for even two whole years—though that's rare. No one is leaving anyone love notes around the house anymore. You find you are fighting with increasing regularity, perhaps so much so that you start to think that the love of your life is no longer the right person for you. You start to wonder if you should break up. Well, the truth of the matter is that if you do, you'll be left the same person you were before her, with only one right leg and one right arm, still searching for a mate with one left leg and left arm who will make you feel whole.

"And what this workshop does is help you and your partner grow your own limbs so that you two can walk side by side as whole individual people, together. And you can do that by . . . well, would you like to read the book?"

"Sure," I said nonchalantly, as if I wasn't absolutely riveted and desperate.

"I'll send it to you tomorrow," he promised.

"Great, thanks," I said, and then asked if they'd like to go in and watch John's next scene.

My first self-help book. It came right away with a note of encouragement:

You make such a great couple. I hope this helps.
All the best,
Craig

I couldn't wait to start reading. Almost immediately, I was surprised that none of my therapists had ever explained relationships to me the way Harville did. *Was he a quack, or was he legitimate?* I wondered. *Or was it just part of the therapeutic process that therapists don't reveal their theories? Would familiarity with theories inhibit therapy?*

According to Harville,

> Most people are attracted to mates who have their caretakers' positive and negative traits, and, typically, the negative traits are more influential . . . and what your old brain was trying to do was re-create the conditions of your upbringing, in order to correct them . . . it was attempting to return to the scene of your original frustration so that you could resolve your unfinished business.

Okay, I thought, *so if I'm attracted to John because he has both positive and negative traits that resemble those of my parents, what are they?* Off the top of my head, I could see some similarities.

Like my dad, John was artistic and ambitious and took risks, but like my mom, he was very concerned with every penny he spent—even more so. And like my mom, he lived in fear of the risks that his partner (me) took. John was funny like my father, always improvising made-up, fun stories with people. And as I saw in San Francisco, John could have a temper like my father used to have when I was growing up. When my dad was finally driven to scream, I became the most frightened I ever was as a child. On the other hand, my father and I really understood each other, similar to the special connection John and I have. And like my mother, John very often wouldn't tell me how he was feeling. Instead he'd act a certain way to me which made me surmise how he/she was feeling (even if I was wrong). And then, of course, John, like my mom, was from Kansas City. Well, okay, Harville, I'm with you so far, I understand that theoretically, according to your "Imago Relationship Therapy," John could be the perfect person for me to be with because he re-creates the conditions of my childhood for me, so now as an adult I can work through the damage my parents unwittingly caused me and grow.

Mmmmm, I thought. Maybe I wasn't avoiding my tracks by dating John like I thought I was. Seems like according to Harville, I was following them more than ever. Did I need a Ph.D. to understand myself/our relationship more accurately? While I was having a hard time synthesizing the different ideas I'd learned from years of therapy with Harville's theories, I was nonetheless filling up with hope.

Harville continued:

The ingredients necessary for full growth and healing—attention, concentration, security, time, deepest intimacy, and the full mirroring of ourselves through our partner—are possible only in marriage. It is through the commitment to accept and heal the other's wounds, to provide a safe haven for the partner to experience his or her wholeness over a lifetime, that we are able to recapture our original wholeness. We cannot heal ourselves, and we cannot heal in open-ended, precarious relationships.

Wow. Commitment to your partner is a prerequisite for healing yourself? I can't heal myself? Even with tons of therapy? Could that be true? You can't grow beyond a certain point alone? I wondered. But it made sense to me that if someone had one foot in and one foot out the door, no progress could be made. I'd just never thought about it before.

Soon John and I were caught in another one of our at-wit's-end fights, me slapping my thighs, dripping in tears, him screaming and walking out the door. It was so bad and I was so worn-out by our lack of progress that I thought, *This is it! Why not just break up? We're both miserable.* But then I re-minded myself of what Harville had said and I thought, *What? Am I going to break up with John only to have to mourn the breakup, reestablish my own life separate from him and his friends, be lonely, start to date, maybe have a few flings with guys who have girlfriends, then feel over-John enough to start looking for someone seriously, then think that I have finally found him only to be dumped and then maybe a year or two later finally find someone I actually fall in love with even though throughout the fall-in-love time I will be anxiety-ridden over the fact that the fun will soon end and then the problems will take over and then I'll find myself having the exact same types of fights that John and I had? Is that what I wanted?* So, I said to myself, *why not just try to work this shit out now? John is willing. He's in therapy with Robert and John wants to be a truly authentic person and a good man. He goes to Alcoholics Anonymous meetings—even though he's not working the steps, at least he's going. And he's willing to try a new couples therapist. And he's a talented, bright, funny guy who loves my work, loves me, has great friends, has an interesting life . . . who else do I think I'm going to find? Of course we have problems, but isn't that what I wanted, someone to work on them with? I have to get my afraid/lazy ass to Al-Anon before I can just give up.*

When I later was back in DLB's office telling her nothing new, I asked her what she thought of John moving out for a limited period of time, to give us space while we worked on our problems.

"Well, that is not a good idea if you truly want to work things out with John. Studies show that if someone moves out, he will more than likely never move back in."

I understood the statistics. If your partner wasn't living with you, the problems weren't as likely to surface and then you wouldn't have as many opportunities to work on them. Also, if John moved out, I might, or he might, find we like our lives fight-free, and not feel the desire to spend time with someone we fight with so often. So I decided I wanted to stay with John. I wanted to forgo all of the breaking up, being lonely, being single and dating, and being on the lookout for someone less troubled only to find myself right back where I was. I decided I wanted to stick it out. I was hoping our new couples therapist, Patti McDonald, was going to be our savior.

thirty-seven
date night

Patti McDonald was so neutral that she wouldn't let either one of us talk about any "us" stuff when one person left to go to the bathroom. Perfect! Now we could really start to make some progress.

By the end of our first session—in response to my complaints that John spent too much time being James Bond killing digital double agents in front of the TV, petting his cat, and talking on the phone for hours when he walked in the door because he didn't want to spend thirty-five dollars a month on a cell phone—Neutral Patti recommended we have a "date night" once a week. That way I'd be guaranteed some just-us time.

Unfortunately, I had to be the one who fucked up our first official therapist-prescribed date night. Forcing myself to become a responsible person who was in a committed relationship with a recovering alcoholic, I finally made myself go to an Al-Anon meeting. I knew I couldn't complain about John's alcoholism to Neutral Patti unless I was doing my part. I'd found an all-women's meeting on Friday at five-thirty that was walking distance from my apartment, and made myself go.

My heart was pounding as I walked in the door to the little room in the church's basement. A number of the women smiled or said hello as I found a seat. I wanted to look at some literature on the literature table but wasn't dying to advertise my newcomer status. I didn't want to talk to anyone, I just wanted to be invisible. The meeting got under way and I soon found myself grateful for being in a relationship that didn't involve screaming at each other on the roof of a car or getting dragged by my hair down the block like this other rather pulled-together-looking woman was. Some of these women had much more seriously dysfunctional relationships than I did, but encouragingly, many had been able to successfully improve their relationships as well.

As several of the women continued to share their experiences and their knowledge of the program, I started to realize what a major part I played in our screaming/leaving-the-house/returning/screaming/sleeping-on-the-sofa dynamic. If I didn't respond to what John said the way I automatically did, he wouldn't respond to me the way he did. I could take a breath and change my response. I couldn't control him but I could control myself. No one was forcing me to scream and yell and slap my thighs in a rage. I didn't have to let myself get as upset as I usually did just because he had a bad day. We were, in fact, separate people.

It seemed I had little choice but to diagnose myself as "codependent." My happiness depended on John's happiness. My own feelings depended on his feelings. I continually did what Robert's handout called "hooking in."

It was a relief to be learning what I was learning. And I was eager to get home to our date night to tell John how different I was going to be and how much I was doing for our relationship. But I'd miscalculated. I thought the meeting was only an hour, but it was an hour and a half. And I hadn't allowed time for talking to people after the meeting or for the time it would take me to walk home. So, it was a big surprise when I walked in the door for our date night only to find my date upset at me.

"Where have you been? Didn't we have a seven-o'clock date? Wasn't date night what you wanted? The dinner I cooked is cold."

"I'm so sorry, honey, I was at an Al-Anon meeting . . ." I started to say, trying to give him my valid excuse that he didn't think was so valid. I was busy trying to save our relationship by going to Al-Anon while he was busy trying to save our relationship by complying with N.P.'s prescribed date night and going the extra mile by cooking for me. And where did it land us? Fighting. I couldn't believe that all of our self-help efforts were creating more problems than they were solving. We were a joke.

thirty-eight

another successful date night

Early in the day of our next date night, John told me that he had something important that he wanted to talk to me about at dinner. Instantly I was more anxious than curious.

"What is it?" I wanted to know.

"I'll tell you at dinner."

"Is it bad?"

"Don't worry. I'll tell you at dinner."

The setting he chose to tell me the important thing he had to tell me was an almost empty Indian restaurant.

Once we'd settled into our booth and had placed our order, John spoke to me with the gravity and tone he had used with my grandparents the night of our moving-in announcement.

"Honey, I don't know what is wrong with me. And I don't know if I'm ever going to get better. I want you to know that I love you very much and that I need to know that if it turns out that I never get better, if the desire to have sex never comes back, will you leave me?"

It was excruciating to watch John struggle to tell me what he just had to tell me. I couldn't believe that he thought that there was a good chance that he might never want to sex again in his whole life. He was only thirty-three. He'd obviously been suffering a long time and had finally come to an impasse. He wanted desperately to want me and felt so betrayed by his body, even angry at it, for all the problems it was causing our relationship.

As I listened to John, I thought Harville would think that John would never get better unless I committed to him completely. I saw myself as John's salvation. I couldn't leave him because I would doom him to a life of never wanting to fuck beyond wanting to fuck the first few months he was dating someone. And who else in the world was he going to find who was not only so perfect for him in so many ways—interests, humor, ambitions, quirkiness—but who also thought that a bad sex life was a reason to stay with someone, not to leave someone?

"Don't worry, Angelhead, we'll work through this together," I said as I wondered what our life would be like if he never got better. Would we develop an alternative type of sexual relationship like the couple in the Almodóvar film *Live Flesh*, where the paralyzed husband gives his wife head by hoisting her above his head in the bathtub? Would I be expected to not have affairs? Would he want me to? Instead of probing further, I told John, as if I was confident, "Honey, I know you'll get better. I don't believe you'll never want to have sex again. Of course I won't leave you. We'll work through this together."

"But *if* I never get better, will you leave me?" he asked, unwilling to rely on my optimism.

"But I know you'll get better," I said.

"Yes, but if I don't."

"I know you will."

"Yes, but if I don't."

"You will."

"I might not."

"You will."

"I might not."

"I won't leave you, John, because I love you," I finally said, realizing it was what he needed to hear and what Harville thought was necessary.

"I love you," John said, totally relieved.

And then we finished our dinner in silence as I wondered if I had just made a promise I couldn't keep.

thirty-nine

patience for the patient

Soon we graduated from **SCHEDULED DATE NIGHTS** to **SCHEDULED SEXUAL MASSAGE NIGHTS** to **SCHEDULED SEX NIGHTS.** After a modicum of success, things got worse.

We reported to Neutral Patti our more-than-disturbing **SCHEDULED SEX NIGHT** where I found an unresponsive John's eyes glazed over as he lay curled up on the bed trying to be present for an event he had no interest in.

After listening carefully and asking a few probing questions, N.P. said, "John, in my professional opinion, you are clinically depressed and have been for a long time. When you were a practicing alcoholic, you were self-medicating your depression. Does that make sense?"

Taken aback by N.P.'s diagnosis, he nodded.

"Often what happens when an alcoholic first becomes sober is that they feel euphoric. And that can last anywhere from a few weeks to a few years. And then, afterward, that's when depression resets in. I think it would be very helpful for you to take antidepressants in addition to the work you are doing here, with your therapist and in AA."

Still taken aback, John didn't say a thing.

N.P. continued, "There really isn't anything to be afraid

of. It's not like you will feel a drastic change overnight. Rather, you'll gradually feel like a fog has lifted."

I sat there silently. She was making so much sense. John was depressed and now he'd have to face it. Prozac would be our salvation.

Finally, John mustered the strength to ask a question. As it turned out, it was a rather relevant one. "Don't most antidepressants have an adverse effect on one's libido?"

"Not to worry. There have been so many advances in the field of psychopharmacology that there is sure to be something that will help you with your depression without affecting your libido. Or maybe your doctor will recommend you take Viagra to offset the side effects."

John—not dying to go on antidepressants because he associated them with taking whatever non-FDA-approved drugs he'd previously used to help him not feel the terrible way he was feeling—said, "Okay, well, I'll discuss all of this with Robert."

That was the end of the antidepressants discussion for now. Patti introduced the idea and I knew enough to know that I had to be patient, that it would take some time for John to digest the concept, to mull it over, to talk to Robert, to then talk to Patti again, to then eventually get a referral from the insurance company for a psychiatrist, to then make an appointment with the psychiatrist, to go to the appointment to get the prescription, to get the prescription filled, to start the drug, to wait for the drug to kick in, and to finally see if it was the right one for him. But at least I knew he'd follow through. He was a self-diagnosed obsessive-compulsive. If something was on his calendar, it was as good as done. I just had to be patient.

forty

crying yentas

It was Grandmother Honey's eighty-eighth birthday and my mom was throwing her a surprise Sweet Sixteen. After Grandmother was surprised, overwhelmed by it all, and excited about her party, the kibitzing, the oohs and ahhs at the Celebration Booklets I'd made for the party and the seemingly never-ending series of family photos began. Eventually, everyone sat down for lunch as the speeches— the hallmark of our family's events—commenced.

After my mother welcomed everyone and my dad and aunt followed suit, all of the grandchildren, one by one, stood up. After the final applause for my cousin Mark, people started to talk among themselves. But then John stood up and clinked his fork against his glass. After a charming introduction about how Grandmother truly was the star of her own film that he was thrilled to have been cast a part in, he cut right to the chase.

"During Yom Kippur services last year, Honey handed me a brochure about a course on Judaism . . ." Everyone wondered the same thing at the same time: *Was an engagement about to be announced*? All the chattering yentas, who generally thought it okay to talk through a speech as long as they switched to a stage whisper, stopped their not-so-quiet chattering.

John continued, "Well, Honey, I want you to know

that out of respect for you, your family, and my love for your granddaughter, I signed up for that very class last October. My intention was to learn about your religion, never to convert. For six months Jennifer and I went to class every Sunday. We went to temple. I read a lot of books. I learned how to read Hebrew and I celebrated the holidays. And I fell in love with Judaism. The course coincided with a crack in my spiritual door, and a lot of what I learned about Judaism and its love of questions and study greatly appealed to me. I thought this occasion, your eighty-eighth birthday, would be an appropriate time to announce that after a considerable amount of thought, I have recently decided to convert to Judaism. Happy birthday!"

Even though I knew he was going to convert, I had no idea he was going to make this surprise announcement. Tears filled my proud eyes. The yentas were all crying, too. Cheers of "mazel tov" filled the room. He was flooded with hugs until Grandmother interrupted the lovefest by saying, "Noah, we haven't heard from you." Can you imagine having to follow that?

John's day of reckoning soon arrived. After his ritual circumcision (during which the *moyel*, who was to ceremoniously circumsise an already-circumsised John, prattled on about his son's screenplay), John was ready to face the three rabbis for the Bet Din. He answered all of their questions, what this holiday meant, what that one did. Who Moses was, who was Abraham? And why did he want to become a Jew? Impressed across the board, they all signed his he's-a-Jew document. Finally, he went to the *mikvah*, the ritual bath from which he'd emerge a Jew.

My family didn't throw one party; they threw two.

John the Jew. My grandparents gave John a talit and a yarmulke for his conversion. They couldn't have been more proud.

forty-one

good morning

John was in Las Vegas for a typical, debaucherous, not-remotely-his-scene bachelor party for his friend Seth when he found himself at the bar with a guy who had both the same name and the same drink—soda water.

"Are you a friend of Bill's?" this John asked my John.

"Mmm, well, no, I don't think I know a Bill," my John said, as if he hadn't been going to AA meetings for almost three years. He didn't remember that the question was the code recovering alcoholics used to find out if someone was in the program while protecting his anonymity. ("Bill" is Bill W., the founder of Alcoholics Anonymous.) Finally, my John figured out what the other John was saying and said yes.

The two Johns got to talking and the conversation changed my life. By the end of the weekend, the other John had invited my John to his "home" meeting, a very serious men's stag AA meeting in Westwood. Reluctantly, John agreed to go the following week, not wanting to hurt the guy's feelings.

It was because of this soon-to-be-life-altering AA meeting that John realized how unrecovered he really was. He couldn't fuck his girlfriend, who he was afraid would soon leave him. He lived in fear of being a broke failure. He was afraid of people not liking him. His whole life was guided by/motivated by fear. He was desperately unhappy. Three years after his last drink, he was finally ready to really take step one, to admit that his life had become unmanageable.

So motivated was John that, a couple of meetings later, he bravely asked a nice man named Brent to be his sponsor. Brent would help him "work" the steps. John's secret agenda was to diligently get through them all as soon as possible so that he'd evolve into the person he thought I would want to marry. He naively thought he could just march right through them. He still thought he was in control of his life, not realizing that it was that thinking that landed him in the misery in which he currently dwelled. Clearly he hadn't done such a great job of willing his life where he wanted it to be.

What I didn't know was that part of working the steps involved an incredible amount of self-reflecting and writing. Soon every morning John was writing furiously in his lined notebook. Eventually he was hard at work on his fourth step—taking a "moral and fearless inventory"—writing down all of the people he resented and then exploring why he was upset with them and what he should have done in the same circumstances instead of what he had done. When that was done (two years later), he'd have to take his "sex inventory" by writing down all of the partners he could remember, how he might have harmed them, and what he should have done differently. While I was extremely curious and a notorious snoop, I respected his privacy and didn't open up the journal that he kept on the third shelf of his closet.

Unfortunately for the both of us, I started to resent AA, just as I had this Jewish meditation class he signed up for and the introduction-to-Judaism course before that. All of his reading, meditation, and writing were just more activities that took him away from me. And I knew I couldn't complain about it because these things that were taking him away from me were eventually supposed to deliver him to me. But lying in bed every morning aching for a cuddle, I couldn't help but resent his jam-packed morning routine.

I knew that it was a particularly hard time for him. He'd recently finished the sitcom for the season and had to endure three months of uncertainty while he waited to find out if his contract would be picked up for another year. Meanwhile, the money he'd made afforded him free time. Free time he was determined to not squander. I'd never seen or heard of such a busy morning routine, full of meditating, writing in his meditation journal, reading at least three different books for twenty minutes each (usually a historical novel, a religious text, and a self-help book), responding to e-mails (all of which had to be spell-checked), doing his fourth-step work, and that was all before his shower and cleansing ritual that involved soaps, toners, prescription creams, flossing, and God knows what else. And I felt a lot of feelings about all of this.

One of them was good old-fashioned jealousy. I wanted to be so productive, so motivated, so educated, and so well cared for. Instead I just lay there while John methodically got a fuck load accomplished. But more than that, I was hurt. I was hurt that he could schedule time to do all of that stuff but couldn't manage to schedule two minutes into all of his morning activities to hug, kiss, and squeeze me. All I was asking for was two minutes of loving. While I wanted cuddling to be as much a part of his morning routine as cleaning the cat litter, what I really wanted was for him to want to cuddle, not to cuddle just because it's what I wanted. I felt confident the former could eventually be accomplished but I wondered about the latter.

Meanwhile we got engaged.

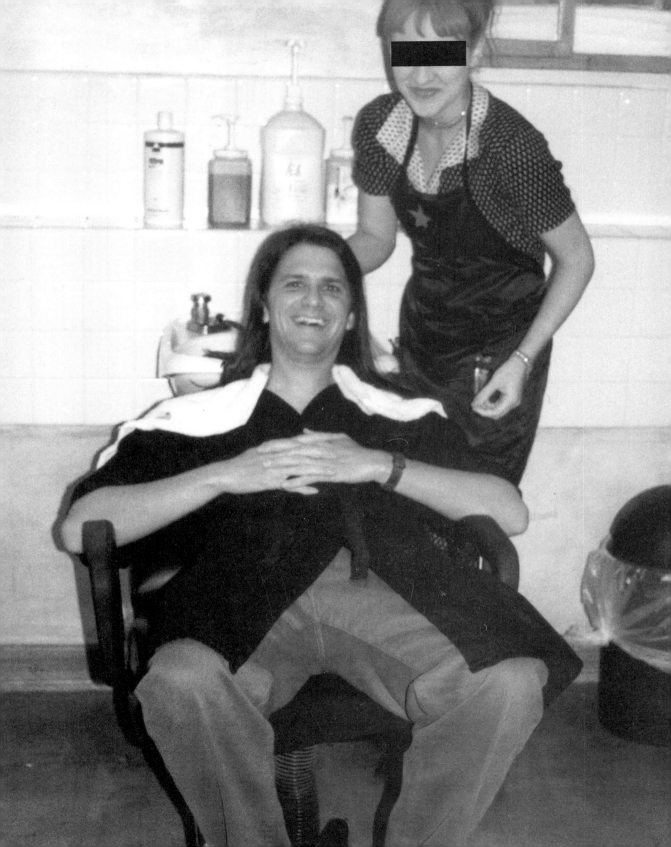

forty-two

yippy skippy

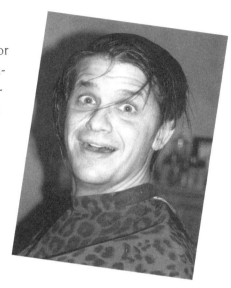

We always said we'd set aside time for our big talk to discuss like two grown-ups the when, why, and hows of getting married. And now somehow we decided that despite the mess we were working hard to get ourselves out of, we were ready for the big talk and wouldn't it be romantic to have it in the woods under the moonlight while we camped for my thirtieth birthday? We weren't saying we were getting married, we were saying we were ready to discuss it. And even though that's officially what we were saying, what we were really saying is that this was it, we were going to do it. Nobody was fooling anybody.

Perhaps subconsciously we thought that "good news" or maybe just "big news" might obliterate John's bad news. He'd recently found out he was definitely not going to be doing another season of the sitcom. Even though he was crammed full of feelings of failure and anxiety about his future, he looked cuter than ever because the moment he heard his contract wasn't being renewed, he'd cut his hair off. My frog had truly morphed into a prince.

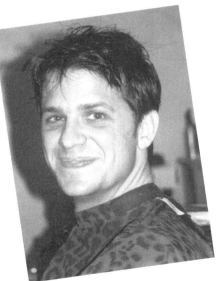

Finally his transformation from frog to prince was complete.

On the way out of town, we stopped by John's storage unit to get his father's 1940s yellow pup tent and all of his camping supplies. A former Boy Scout, John loved camping and was confident the experience would change the skeptical mind of his Jewish princess. We wound up and up and up the Los Angeles Mountains and soon found our turnoff. I had pictured us out in the woods alone, and was surprised to find that our parking space and fire pit were just thirty yards from another family, and another and another and another. A packed campground full of screaming kids wasn't my idea of romantic, but I didn't dwell on it.

John was impressive—totally in his element. He pitched the tent. He attached a rock to the end of a rope and threw it over a tree branch, tying our oil lamp to the other end and hoisting it high. He built the fire. He cooked hot dogs for lunch and made "hobos" for dinner. After eating s'more after s'more, we decided we were ready for *the* talk.

As much as I was against the down-on-the-knee proposal, I still wanted a speech. I wanted to know what John loved about me, why he wanted to get married, and what he thought about marriage. And I wanted to tell him what I thought—hoping that in the telling I would actually *really* think about it for once. I'd been so consumed by our dramas, and so distracted by my feminist views on the "right" way to get engaged, that I never truly thought about if I was ready and/or even interested in getting married. So now I was hoping we'd come to some kind of consensus together. But we didn't. We just jumped right in. We did a you-first-no-you-first-okay-I'll-go-first thing, which resulted in John going first.

Sitting on a log, John simply turned to me and said, "Jennifer, will you marry me?"

Giving him a second to add something more onto his proposal, perhaps something about how I was the most this and the most that and that he couldn't live without me, I paused for a moment. And then, after I realized he had nothing more to say, I said, "Yes."

Then John smiled at me and waited for my question.

"Will you marry me?" I said, hoping I'd find the courage to say more, but I didn't.

"Yes," he said and then he leaned over to kiss me.

John was more affectionate with me that night than he had been in a long time. And while I reveled in the attention, I was plagued with a sense of dissatisfaction and unease. I told myself that this is what I got for being so anti the surprise proposal. Perhaps women craved them so much because they forced usually uncommunicative men to articulate their love in a big-enough way that the impact would last for a good long while. But hadn't I made it clear that we should talk about getting married before jumping right into the proposal? Where was the discussion? *Just say, "Wait, honey, let's talk about this some more,"* I encouraged myself. *Why am I letting this happen so fast?* Despite all of my questions, I didn't say a word.

We went to bed that night in our tent and like good young engagers in love we fucked, or at least we tried to. With a rock digging into my back, his hands went down my pants and I came and I sucked him and I sucked him and he didn't come and then I needed to pee and returned to a fiancé who said we didn't have to try anymore. And then throughout the night, I had to get up four more times to pee, which was a total pain in the ass and turned me against camping for good. The next morning, we took a beautiful long walk, enjoyed the great outdoors, and left.

We decided to keep the engagement to ourselves and officially announce it in a month and a half when the family got together for Rosh Hashanah, which was also Grandpa's birthday. Keeping our intentions a secret was a relief because I didn't feel like announcing anything to anyone. I was hoping we'd be in better shape by the time the holiday rolled around. Meanwhile I went ring shopping. Guilt-free shopping for expensive things— my favorite activity.

The following Tuesday, we reported our news to Neutral P.

"Congratulations!"

"Thank you," we said.

"So how does it feel? Do you feel yippy skippy?" she asked, noticing the lack of overjoyedness on our faces.

We smiled. But no, I said, I did not feel yippy skippy for God's sake. John was a depressed, just-starting-to-recover alcoholic who adhered to ridiculously strict schedules and didn't tell me why he wanted to marry me and our sex life still sucked. She knew that. She also knew I was a too-old-to-be-dependent-on-my-parents woman who was attracted to a depressed, just-starting-to-recover alcoholic who had a decent amount to do with the fact that our sex life sucked. Of course I didn't feel yippy skippy.

forty-three

if i understand what you're saying correctly

Neutral P. could plainly see that when we recounted a fight from earlier in the week, earlier in the month, or earlier in the year, we relived it. It was always as if no time had passed, as if we hadn't been getting along just fine for the past six days because there we were, back at it, defending our positions and blaming the other with fervor. I'd want nothing more than to prove to N.P. that the way I said it happened was *the* definitive way that it happened. I wasn't to blame, John was. If he could only understand what really happened, he wouldn't feel the wrong way he was feeling about it. And poor John, who didn't have as sharp a memory for the details of the way things happened as I did, resented the way I'd just throw out facts as if they were irrefutable. Was I really right? Could I always be right? If so, why did he feel so differently about what had happened?

N.P. pointed out that it seemed to her that I cared a lot more about being right than about how John felt. Even though I was clearly smart enough to always defend myself against any accusations of wrongdoing, relationships weren't about right and wrong. Her office wasn't a courtroom. Being right had nothing to do with understanding, compassion, compromise, or love. I was always in a state of defending my case or prosecuting it instead of learning about why we might feel so differently about the same event.

Without announcing it, N.P. was changing her approach. Instead of focusing on sex—when to schedule it, who should control it—she was going to focus on our communication, hoping improvement in the latter would lead to improvement in the former. Looking back, I think that was the route Robert was trying to take before it blew up in our faces.

Neutral P. said that we needed to learn to listen to each other and care about the way the other person perceives a situation even if we don't agree with it. The first step was for each person to truly feel that the other person understood his/her point of view.

"Whenever you find yourselves fighting about something, about anything, the first thing I want you to do is to stop and agree on a time to come back and discuss it. At a minimum it should be twenty minutes because that is how long it takes for the body's physiology to change from one emotional state to another. Pursuing the discussion while you are both worked up will be very difficult and most certainly fruitless. Now, once you return to have the discussion, one of you will go first.

"For the purpose of explanation, let's say it's Jennifer. First, Jennifer, you tell John—from start to finish—your version of the course of events and how you felt along the way. John, it is your job to listen. You cannot interrupt Jennifer to clarify or defend your position. You will soon have your turn. When Jennifer is completely finished, John, it is your turn to say back to Jennifer what she just told you. A helpful way to start is to say, 'If I understand what you're saying correctly . . .' " explained Neutral P.

"Then," N.P. continued, "Jennifer sits quietly and listens to John's rendition of what she just said. Jennifer, if you disagree with John's interpretation at any point, do not interrupt. You will have your turn. Just hear John out. Then, when John is finished, you can clarify for him which parts you think he didn't understand. When she is finished, John, it is then your turn to say back to Jennifer what you just heard.

"You are to go back and forth like this until Jennifer feels that her position is entirely understood by John, even if he disagrees with it entirely. That is not what is important at this point. Then, when Jennifer is entirely satisfied, it is John's turn to give his version of the events. You will then repeat the same process entirely until John feels entirely understood. What is most important is to understand and to feel understood—not to be right or to win the argument."

And so right there in front of Neutral Patti, for the next hour or so, we practiced communicating the way she wanted us to. We tried her system out on a fight we'd had over a left turn I had made coming out of the airport's Parking Lot C a couple of months ago. The fight was so terrible that it had instantly rendered our relaxing, fun vacation a waste of money. We had ended up hating each other before we walked into our front door.

John began. And it was incredible. For the first time I understood why he responded the way he had (which had initially infuriated me) because I saw it through his eyes. And I felt so sympathetic and frustrated toward me on his behalf. And then I went and he felt the same way. We were shocked by how well Neutral Patti's if-I-understand-what-you're-saying-correctly way of communicating worked. Not only did it restore my confidence in N.P., it was the most liberating experience of my life.

We quickly became Mr. and Mrs. If-I-understand-what-you're-saying-correctly. We clung to those let's-calm-this-situation-the-fuck-down words with our life because they were in fact our lifesavers. We practiced all the time.

forty-four

engaging

As engagers we had to have the proper engagement accoutrements. John bought me a vintage ring of my choice and I bought him a vintage watch of his. The only thing we had left to do was announce our intentions. With Rosh Hashanah/Grandpa's birthday a few weeks away, the clock we didn't have to listen to was ticking. Our communication progress was making me feel better about our engagement—though I was yet to be without reservations. It's not like we were screwing again. But we were fighting a lot less ever since we'd been "understanding more of what each other was saying correctly." Perhaps it was also the buffer of the long engagement we both wanted that allowed me to feel pretty good about something I wasn't entirely sure I was happy about. I reasoned that surely after another year and a half of couples therapy, AA, and John's new antidepressants (which he'd *finally* just started), we would have improved enough for me to feel good about committing to spend my life loving John and only John.

So there we were, all singing "Happy Birthday" to Grandpa—the lead-in for the usual round of speeches. The room was at full capacity as the twelve people from the breakfast room came to stand in the dining room, joining the other twenty of us. After my dad's toast and my mom's poem, I passed out a song sheet. I had written a version of Queen's "We Are the Champions," personalized for Grandpa. I asked everyone to join me in the chorus. After the applause, John stood up and said he had something to say as I left my post next to Grandpa at the head of the table and walked over to join him in the middle of the room.

Wearing his sixties-style dark green suit that I had picked out at a vintage store the day before we had to go to an acquaintance's wedding—another friend's marriage that had already ended in divorce—John looked very handsome. I was nervous as hell and grateful to have a fiancé who was not only so well-spoken, funny, and comfortable in front of a crowd, but one who could pull this off with all of the pomp, circumstance, and panache it deserved. We had a love of pomp and circumstance in common.

John started by recalling the dinner when he told my grandparents that we were going to be living together.

"As some of you may know, Jennifer and I went out to dinner with Honey and Julius about nine months ago. The purpose of the dinner was to tell them that we had decided to move in together. Now, as some of you may also know, this is not something that Honey and Julius necessarily approve of. And so I wanted to explain to them in person why we were doing it."

Now some people in the room were starting to think, *Hey, wait, is this about Grandpa or about something else? Could it be?*

"Now I am here to report that Grandpa Julius is more open-minded than some of you might think."

Oh, okay, everyone thought, *this actually is about Grandpa.*

"And while he was understanding of our reasons, he nonetheless said that this 'living-together business' couldn't go on forever and that we should make a decision by his eighty-eighth birthday."

Jesus Christ, all the Jews thought, *it really is happening.*

"Now, while I want you all to know that I have a great deal of respect for Julius, Jennifer and I certainly didn't want to decide something as important as marriage on someone else's clock, *even* if it is Grandpa Julius's."

This was more than the group could take. People were simply too

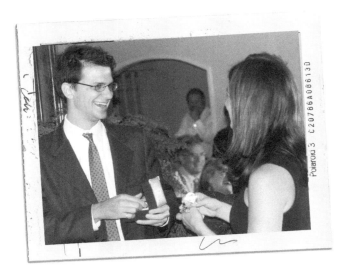

I said yes and then he said yes, and then finally, this time we did feel yippy skippy.

nervous to make any nervous laughter audible. Meanwhile, John couldn't have enjoyed milking it more than he was.

"However," John continued, "it just so happened that our desire to take the next step"—the hearts in the room started to beat faster again—"just happened to coincide with Julius's birthday. And that in front of all of our friends and family I'd like to say that I love Jennifer very much." And then he took the ring box out of his pocket and opened it up to a chorus of gasps just as I took out the watch box. We opened them simultaneously and then we turned toward each other.

"Jennifer, will you marry me?"

"Yes, John, will you marry me?"

"Yes, I will," he said, and then we kissed and hugged, our smiles beaming right off our faces as everyone burst into applause, cheers, and tears. We made our way through the crowd, hugging everyone as the mazel tovs and congratulations and when's-the-weddings and I-want-to-throw-the-showers ensued. John and I went home excited by our news and how well we'd performed it.

It wasn't long before my mother's best friend told me that while my mother was very excited about the wedding, she wasn't so pleased with the year-and-a-half-away date we'd chosen. Soon my mother would tell me herself.

"Jennifer, Dad and I couldn't be more pleased that you and John are getting married. And while I would never in my life rush along a couple who was thinking about getting engaged, now that you have already made the decision, I don't see why you have to wait so long to get married. Your grandparents are getting very old and the truth is we just don't know how their health will be in a year and a half—that is, if they are even alive. And I know they would just love to feel well for such an important event."

"Mother, Grandma and Grandpa aren't even sick. They are just fine. I just don't see why we should change what we think is right for us based on something that might happen to them," I explained, not using my most respectful, patient voice.

I didn't budge on my position and we ended the conversation with my mom still frustrated by our decision. While she probably thought I was being selfish and stubborn, I wondered if she wondered why I might be behaving that way.

My compelling reasons to have some significant amount of time before the wedding were the exact things that I would never have told my mother in a million years. I could never have said, "Mom, to tell you the truth, I want more time to feel better about our relationship before we get married. I have a certain confidence that I will, so if you'll just bear with me." That would certainly beg the question, "Oh my goodness, honey, what kind of things do you want to feel better about and why did you get engaged if you have reservations?" And while I never would have said the above in a million years, I never would have answered the question with the truth in a gagillion years, "Well, Mom, John and I have a terrible sex life. John's afraid he might not want to have sex again. John is depressed and I'm oppressive. And I want to make sure he loves me and adores me and finds me attractive in ways that would give me the confidence to want to spend my life with him. We need as much time as we can get."

forty-five
good luck to me

John and I planned an engagement party for our friends in New York at my parents' apartment. The day of, we were hanging out when we suddenly found ourselves going at it on the sofa—me on top enduring full-on knee burn, thinking, *When we finally do it, does it have to be so fast and frenzied*? *Where is the quiet, I-love-you-sweetheart-and-am-thrilled-to-be-marrying-you sex* I *was hoping for*? It's not like I was against fast and furious, it's just that as the one sex encounter in a long time, and certainly as a new engager, I was longing for something more sensual, more LOVING.

Back in L.A., at our next couples-therapy session, John proudly reported to Neutral Patti that we had had sex in New York. In an effort to be honest, just so N.P. didn't get the wrong impression, I told her that while it's true we did do it, it wasn't so great.

John was devastated. He couldn't win. I was impossible to please. Unpleasable. Here he was doing everything he could—working the steps, taking antidepressants, going to therapy, going to the urologist, going to couples therapy, talking in if-I-understand-what-you're-saying-correctlys, *and* fucking me—and I still wasn't happy. If things didn't go just as I wanted, I was unhappy, which means I would always be unhappy.

N.P. had to agree with John.

"Jennifer, there is some validity to what John is saying. I think you have a real tendency to see the glass as half empty."

I felt terrible that I had made John feel like he couldn't win for trying. I mean who would want to fuck me when it seems that I have such exacting standards about how I want it done? Be more gentle. Be more loving. Be more aggressive. Who could keep up? I was sooooo mad at myself. I realized that by opening my stupid big mouth that I had single-handedly just sent us back to square one. Here he was finally fucking me and I had to go and say it wasn't a perfect fuck, so now he won't dare fuck me again for a good long while because first he'll have to get over this and then he'll have to regain trust in me. Fuuuuuck. I apologized profusely, but I knew it wasn't enough.

A couple of months later, I found myself still paying for how glass-half-emptied I'd been about our frenzied pre-engagement-party sex. Hadn't I been paying for that thoughtless fuck-up long enough? I wondered if John was secretly relieved that I'd fucked up the way I had because it actually bought him some time to not have to think about having to do it. *What the fuck was I doing marrying a man whom I'd barely fucked over the past year or so?*

John, too, was at wit's end. He even said he thought that it was almost laughable that we were getting married when we still weren't having sex. We were both devastated by our predicament and felt trapped. We'd been in couples therapy for almost a year, and while our communication had certainly improved, our sex life had gotten worse—if that was possible! We simply had stopped having sex. No sex at all.

N.P. had a new theory.

About an hour after we had what I thought was bad sex and what John thought was fun sex, we were welcoming our guests at our New York engagement party. Two weeks later, I'd complain about it in couples therapy and set us back even further. A photo is not quite worth the thousand words it's cracked up to be.

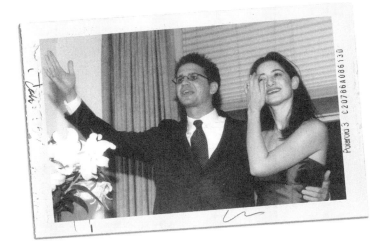

229

"Perhaps we've been focusing our efforts too much on John—which is not to say that we didn't need to address his depression. However, it seems to me that while Jennifer seems to be saying that she is the one who is always willing to have sex, that has been a safe position for her to take because John's depression was having such a strong effect on his libido. It might be that John's situation has given Jennifer license to be very eager for sex because the coast was clear. It was safe. It wouldn't be happening, so she could crave all she wanted. However, now that John is doing so much better, perhaps Jennifer's fears are coming to the fore. Jennifer, remember how critical you were about the sex you had in New York? That only served to alienate you two, not bring you together."

She was right and I knew it.

"Jennifer," she continued, "do you have any sense of what you're afraid of?"

"Well, right off the bat, no. But I can see what you're saying. I mean, at least intellectually, it makes sense," I said, not wanting to have to sit there and go over every one of my mortifying sexcapades and failed relationships.

Of course, John was relieved to hear Patti's latest assessment. He was sick and tired of him always being the one with the problem. Enough of him being depressed. Him being an alcoholic. His Propecia. (It turned out that a second opinion from another urologist did view Propecia as part of the problem and said that it would take his body perhaps nine months or more to adjust to the drug.) Him not wanting to do it. The spotlight was now on me.

I left the session promising Neutral P. I'd think about what she'd said. And I did. I started once again to really think about my past relationships through the lens of a fear of intimacy. I was surprised by how easy it was to do.

Perhaps it was precisely Mickey's, Derek's, and Miknos's heaviness that made me feel safe enough to get close to them in the first place. Perhaps I subconsciously thought their weight gave me an "out" . . . as if fat was a valid reason not to get involved with someone. Subconsciously, I knew I'd never seriously consider a "relationship" with them, so they were okay to get close to for the time being because I wasn't at risk of getting too close.

Perhaps I was able to get excited enough to have my first orgasm with sophomore Pete precisely because of the clothes we wore, the lack of kisses we gave, and the boyfriend/girlfriend status we didn't have.

And perhaps it wasn't such a coincidence that I'd kept my relationship with Dylan very only-lunch until just a month before school was out. Maybe it wasn't a coincidence that I chose to be with a college senior who wouldn't be coming back to school the next year. Maybe it wasn't a coincidence that I chose a man whose father was so close to death that he had to leave school twice to be with him during the one and only month we actually dated. And then, taking it even one step further, maybe I found a level of comfort in being with a man who was so desperately in need of love and support while his father was dying that he was willing to overlook our sex problems just to have the companionship and love I gave him. And the bricks kept falling.

Auggie wasn't fat. He didn't have bad skin. He didn't live across the country. His father wasn't dying. He was a really great-looking, kind, gentle person who wanted to be with me. Of course I didn't wipe well. My subconscious was so desperate to keep me from being intimate that in its eleventh-hour desperation, it managed to successfully pull a this-cannot-happen trick out of a hat.

And so it must be that my fear of intimacy is what caused me to change my feelings about Stuart once he'd finally declared his love for me. After all, all summer long I had pined for his attention. And then the minute he showed up on my doorstep in New York, ready to love me, I found myself repulsed by him. For God's sake, he hadn't changed a bit. It was me and my fear.

And then, of course, we all already knew why I'd been so attracted to so many men who were in love with someone else. That theory supported this fear of intimacy theory.

N.P. was absolutely right. I was very comfortable feeling desire for John because the coast was clear.

I wondered if my fear of intimacy came from something that happened in my upbringing. Or were human beings simply afraid of being close to another because they were afraid of the pain of being left? After all, death would at some point take our loved ones away from us. And wouldn't detachment lessen the pain? I mean, who the hell *wasn't* afraid of intimacy? It seemed to me that virtually every one of my friends was, although they more than likely wouldn't agree.

Just when I was starting to make some real sense of my life, I went to see the Notorious DLB and was surprised when she didn't agree with Neutral P! On the contrary, DLB thought I had a healthy sex drive and that John indeed did account for the majority of our problems. Yes, perhaps I was too clingy and controlling, but John was the one without the drive. Perhaps if I had mustered the courage to share with DLB all of my embarrassing past sexual experiences and my new take on them, she might've agreed with me and N.P. But I didn't. I still liked hearing that our sex problems were mainly John's problem. I liked it, because I was afraid of it being my problem and how that meant I'd have to change.

DLB laid down my options as she saw them.

"In some ways, I think you and John get along brilliantly." She prefaced it with that. "The way I see it is that you can either stay with John and get a 'paramour' "—that's the word she used and it sounded somewhat exciting to me as I started to envision myself sleeping with the guy from yoga I had a crush on—"and John and you can exist like brother and sister, just continuing about your business living under the same roof, or you can try a new approach."

"Well, I'll try anything."

"Okay, well, as an experiment with a time limit, let's say for a period of a month, you are not to have any expectations of cuddling, affection, or sex. None at all. At the same time, however, it is very important that you don't withdraw from John"—like I sometimes did to punish him for not giving me the love, attention, and sex I wanted. "You should do your best to remain your exuberant, loving self."

"What do you mean? I should be loving but not affectionate?"

"I think a helpful way to look at it is to treat John as you would your gay friend Jason. Pretend that Jason has moved in for a month. I know that you hold hands with Jason and give him hugs, but there is no sexual attention and, most importantly, no expectation of reciprocation. While there are no guarantees, this experiment may help alleviate undue pressure on John as well as provide some relief for you."

I drove home wondering if I really would be able to treat John as if he was my gay best friend? *For a whole month*? Well, I was going to try.

forty-six

making marriage work: sex

My trying-to-act-like-John-was-gay experiment ended long before the month was up due to my inability to sustain any serious change in my behavior. And the experiment, or my inability to stick with it, never got a thorough evaluation from the Notorious DLB because another crisis or series thereof took over our sessions. But the experiment did, at least for a short while there, lift the rage out of my body.

It used to be that at bedtime, when I was withholding affection in an attempt to punish John for not loving me enough, in an effort to show him what it feels like to be unkissed and unadored, I'd turn over and go to sleep at the edge of the bed to create as big a gap between us as I could muster. I'd face the closet and wonder if he even noticed. And I'd stew. *Fuck him. Fuck him for not rolling over and spooning me. Fuck him for not playing with my hair. Fuck him for needing space to air out. Fuck him for not hoisting me on top of him for a passionate fuck.* But with DLB's new plan, I had an excuse to let my anger go. I could kiss him and say good night and not expect anything—in the way of a kiss or a hug or an intertwine, let alone an intercourse—and not be upset about it because I was doing it toward a goal and I'd only be doing it for a month. With my rage levels decreasing, I felt lighter and we got along better. John, it seemed, was feeling less suffocated by me and my unrelenting neediness. If you saw us in the latest class we'd signed up for—Making Marriage Work—you probably would have thought we were a particularly happy, self-aware, well-adjusted, in-love couple.

Making Marriage Work was led by a marriage and family therapist who looked like a cross between Rapunzel and one of Snow White's dwarfs because her curly hair was way too long for her short, stocky frame. After her opening remarks, she asked the class—a circle of ten couples—to introduce ourselves and state if we were single, engaged, or married.

"Hello, I'm Heidi."

"And I'm Brent, we just got engaged last month. We haven't set a date yet."

"Uh, yeah, um, I'm Paul."

"And I'm Francine and our wedding is October twenty-second."

And then we came to Melanie and Steve. First she said her name and then he said his and then, at the exact same time, she said "single" and he said "engaged."

"Well, which is it?" we all wanted to know as we laughed and shook our heads.

Turning the back of her hand toward the group and wiggling her fingers, Melanie proved her single status and said, "I don't have a ring."

We all agreed with her. They were not engaged.

"Well, we've been shopping for one," Steve said, sticking up for himself.

"Looking isn't the same as buying!" she snapped back.

"But we just bought a house together," he said, as if a house were a wedding date.

I loved it.

Doc R. handed us all MMW notebooks with the syllabus and readings. The intro read in part:

> We learn about marriage informally, by observing our parents, other family members, and married friends. Parents, our most important tutors, often are not the best examples of marital success . . .

We'd soon find out that with each of the ten couples, one person in the couple had parents who were married, the other had parents who were divorced. The destabilized were looking for some stability.

In contrast to the lack of formal instruction in marital skills, we spend years being trained to be plumbers, teachers, physicians, geologists, or workers in whatever field we select. Yet two of the most important areas of our lives—marriage and parenting—are left to chance!

I couldn't have agreed more. Why did we have to take a driver's license test but no marriage license test? I wondered what the rate of spousal abuse was compared to injuries from auto accidents.

As usual, I was the most vocal in our class. One day I helped clarify for my confused classmates what Doc R. meant when she tried to explain Harville's theory of relationships. Clearly surprised by my succinct and much more understandable explanation, she generously thanked me for my help. Additionally, John was the first to call other guys out on their defensiveness—which surprised the hell out of them. They seemed to expect John to take their side, not point out the weakness of their position. Doc R. couldn't believe how "self-actualized" we were. Even though we were flattered, we knew we weren't self-actualized at all. If we were, wouldn't we be fucking each other? No, we were just a hell of a lot more aware of our problems than anyone else in the class. Instead of getting into anything, we simply replied, "Well, we've had a lot of couples therapy."

I anxiously awaited the sixth class. The subject? Sex. It began with Doc R. handing out minipencils and small pieces of paper. First we were to write down the number of times we'd like to have sex a week. Then, below that, we were to write down the number of times we actually had sex a week.

What a stupid bitch, I'd thought. *Not everybody has sex at least once a week. She should know that. She should have said, "How many times a month?" Way to make people feel bad.* So I wrote down .5 even though at that point it was more like .25—if at all. I was fuming: A *fucking week*?

Then we all folded our little papers and put them in the basket that was being passed around. When it got back to Doc R., she reached in and started reading out the numbers. Most of the top numbers were 2 or 3, with an occasional 4. Most of the bottom numbers were 1 until, of course, she got to my .5, at which point she just stood there wondering out loud what .5 could possibly mean, smiling an inappropriate smile.

What do you think it means, bitch? I thought. *Do you think someone's trying to say the guy's dick is only going halfway into his fiancée's vagina?* Even though the whole exercise was about being anonymous, about not exposing your partner, I couldn't fucking let it go. I blurted out, "Once every two weeks?" in a semi-questioning tone, trying to make it seem like it wasn't *us* that didn't fuck every week, but rather that I was just smarter than she was. However, I don't know if my tone accomplished that. I'm sure everyone knew it was us. Someone else, however, did write zero. So that was a relief. Until later, when I found it was John.

I, of course, had eagerly read the workbook sheets on the topic. One worksheet, "How It All Started" began with a quote from the Hebrew Bible:

"For it is not good that a person be alone . . . and therefore a man leaves his father and his mother and clings to his wife so that they become one flesh." This passage acknowledges the human need for companionship, the primacy of the couple relationship over all others, and the desirability of sex, the merging of two into "one flesh."

If that is the case, I wondered, *why did Jacob—the father of the twelve tribes of Israel—have sex with four women?* Where is the "primacy of the couple relationship" when you're having sex with two sisters—your barren wife, Rachel, and her sister, Leah—as well as with the slave wives of those two sisters? Are you not becoming "one flesh" with the slave wives you are sleeping with if it's your wife who gave them to you to sleep with? Was Rachel's inability to produce offspring excuse enough to forgo the "primacy of the couple"? I wanted a religion that didn't contradict itself. I read on:

In contrast to the early Christians, who insisted that asceticism and celibacy are the purest and holiest life practice, Judaism has always stressed the union of the body and soul of humans, both of which are created by God. Therefore, the pleasures of this world, including sex, are considered God's gifts, to be enjoyed to the fullest.

To me, that was pressure. God *wants* us to be enjoying sex and we're not.

"Not only is sex desirable, but it is holy, when sanctified in a caring, committed relationship . . . It is ordained by God Himself as the means for the perpetuation of the human race and for the ultimate expression of human love," says Rabbi Maurice Lamm.

I've never had holy sex before, I thought. *I've never had ultimate-expression-of-love sex before either.* Back when John and I were fucking, we'd have what I might call good sex, sexy sex, fun sex, and even some loving sex, but I think I can safely say that we had not had this ultimate-expression-of-love sex. *When are we going to ultimately express our love by having sex? How are we ever going to do that?*

Rabbi Lamm says, "The Bible conceives of sex within marriage as the woman's right and the man's duty . . ."

More fuel for my I-deserve-to-be-properly-screwed fire, I thought.
I flipped through the worksheets and found other sex topics like: Early Life Factors That Affect Sexual Response; Biochemical, Hormonal, and Gender Influences on Sexual Response; Social and Psychological Components; Environmental Distractions; Health; Schedules; Stress and Unrealistic Expectations. And then I came to a topic of particular interest: Newlyweds Speak Out About Sex.

Today's couples are far more realistic about their sexual expectations. Because they are better informed and more experienced, they know how to achieve a fulfilling sex life.

More informed, yes, more experienced, yes, but I would have to say I disagree with her conclusion that those factors translate into knowing more how to "achieve a fulfilling sex life." If this Dr. Sylvia Weisshaus was talking about knowing how to get myself and John off, well, yes, but she couldn't be equating that with a fulfilling sex life . . . so either I'm not "typical" or I'm stupid . . . if I understand what she's saying correctly.

> In short, newlyweds today are able to enjoy sex without the worries about how it "ought" to be that often plagued couples in other times . . .

I thought Sylvia was naively optimistic. I thought that surely there are a lot of people out there who are still—in this day and age—plagued by how they think their sex life ought to be. I was among them. Wouldn't this section in the Making Marriage Work packet not need to be included if the situation were as she described it?

And then the dreaded chapter on Sexual Decline:

> One study indicated that almost everything—jobs, commuting, housework, money worries—conspires to reduce sexual interaction, while nothing leads to increasing it. However, it's more the quality of sex that matters now, rather than the quantity . . . because we make love less often, there is more intensity, more depth of feeling, to our intimate moments.

I turned the page but couldn't find the next section that was sure to follow a section on a "Decline in Sex in a Marriage"—that is, a section that addresses how to handle your desire to fuck the mailman while your spouse is stressed out, busy with his career, commuting, and/or doing housework. I kept flipping but found nothing.

forty-seven

making marriage work: money

The course carried on for the next few weeks and I found almost all of it endlessly fascinating. The only thing I was dreading was the last class. The class led by a CP fucking A. The financial-planning class.

At the beginning of our second-to-last class, Doc R. said she wanted to spend the last half hour starting some dialogue about money to prepare us for our last session. When that half hour rolled around, she walked over to the chalkboard, picked up a piece of chalk, and asked, "What does money symbolize?"

As we called out answers, she jotted them down on the board.

SUCCESS

POWER   CONTROL

VALUES

TASTE

John called out,   FREEDOM

Then Doc R. asked a series of questions designed to highlight the effect money can have on a relationship: "How do you as a couple decide how and when to spend your money? Do you both like to spend your money on the same things, like trips, clothes, home furnishings, or appliances? Does the person making more money decide how money is spent?" As she kept firing off the questions, I sat there hating my life, dreading next week's class. Of course we had some homework to do to prepare ourselves for it. We had some worksheets to fill out to make us look at our relationship to money and how the way we were brought up influenced it. We had to answer questions about how similarly or differently our parents each dealt with money. And so for the first time, John and I set out to spell it out for ourselves and then to share it with each other. This is what we came up with:

John had a middle-class upbringing in a suburban town in Kansas. His father was an entrepreneur in the computer business in the seventies and eventually made some real money. He was the first Lehr to do so. Eventually he got bored with his successful company and sold it. His new venture wasn't as successful but nonetheless he believed in it and decided, without telling his wife, to gamble everything on it. Everything included taking out several mortgages on the house, not paying his employees' FICA and Social Security, and of course, the coup de grâce, not paying his own income tax. Suffice to say, he lost everything. And that everything was lost right in front of his two sons' faces. John and his brother were playing basketball in the driveway when the sheriff came to repossess both the new Mercedes and the VW Rabbit. Their "better life" was very short-lived.

Unable to convince her husband to get a real job when he was convinced he could start another successful company, John's mother worked hard to pay back the IRS. She was a social worker by day and at night took in as many typing jobs as she could to supplement her income. She also never bought herself a thing. John's mother never trusted his father again. No trust. No affection. Resentment galore. Divorce. (And of course, that's just the short-short of it.)

By answering the questions on the handout, John realized that because of his father, he didn't trust success. Like his mother, he was desperately afraid of being broke. Afraid of having everything taken away from him. Of spending money on anything unessential. Of having his dreams/life taken away from him to pay off someone else's debt, someone to whom he was legally bound! On the other hand, John had his father in him. John was a dreamer. He wanted to be a big success on his own terms. Inside of him the mother/father war raged.

Unfortunately for John and his issues with money, he was engaged to someone with expensive tastes and a serious credit-card debt to prove it. Someone with an *entirely* different financial background. Someone who had two parents with entirely different and often conflicting relationships to money. Here's what I wrote on my questionnaire:

> *My mother and dad relate to money in very different ways. In this respect, I am more like my dad and John is more like my mom, which is surprising considering that my upper-middle-class upbringing was closer to that of my mom's while John's was more like my dad's.*
>
> *My dad wanted to create a better life for himself than the one he grew up with and as far as I can remember he has always had expensive tastes. My dad loves nice clothes, beautiful cars, great art, and travel. My mom on the other hand is not a shopper, which is not to say she doesn't always like to look appropriate and doesn't enjoy the trips my father plans, but she doesn't crave them. I remember my grandpa telling me that when he'd visit my mom at college she'd declined his gifts of money. He also told me that when he sent her a batch of dresses he'd bought for her in Paris, she chose one and sent the rest back. This was a person I couldn't relate to. I was the opposite, always trying to get my grandparents to buy me something new. I could understand why John worried about money, but could never fully grasp why my mother was similarly plagued.*

Looking at my mother's relationship to money, I wondered how her parents' relationship to it had affected her life and if she'd ever thought about it before. Whatever it was, I got conflicting message from my parents. From my mother, I periodically got that we were in serious financial shape and that the situation required constant monitoring. From my father, I understood that we were rich.

DLB, I recalled, thought my irresponsible approach to my money (i.e., never balancing my checkbook) was a form of rebellion against my mother's obsession with it. I only had one life to live and I didn't want to waste it adding and subtracting numbers as if my life depended on it. But I took my rejection of my mother's approach to money to an unhealthy extreme.

After John and I read our results to each other, I thought of how well we fit into Harville's theory that "people are attracted to mates who have their caretakers' positive and negative traits," how we were attracted to each other because subconsciously we were "attempting to return to the scene of [our] original frustration so that we can resolve [our] unfinished business." John and I were perfect for each other because we gave each other the opportunity to improve our unhealthy relationships to money by working through our differences. If I married someone who was rich and just gave me everything I thought I wanted, would I ever grow and become a responsible adult who actually felt self-sufficient and proud of my work? If John married someone who was equally self-denying and perpetually afraid of the worst, would he ever learn to enjoy life?

Even though I'd prepared for our last class, I still dreaded the hell out of it. In fact I dreaded it so much that I do not remember a thing about it. Well, almost nothing. I remember clearly that I was the only asshole in the class without a full-time job, who wasn't pulling in any income to speak of. Embarrassed by lack of success, I made it seem like I was doing okay, what with my Celebration Books business and my (new) side interior-design job. I sounded impressive and felt like a fraud. I had made two thousand dollars on one booklet job and was making thirty-five an hour (but only like two hundred a week) helping my sister's friend rearrange her apartment and make a few purchases at Pottery Barn.

The CPA handed us a stapled packet with a *Los Angeles Times* article on top called "Test of Your Fiscal Compatibility":

> If you are planning to wed, you'd be wise to find out if you are as in sync fiscally as you are emotionally. Financial conflicts figure into the bulk of serious marriage woes . . . If you have serious differences or find it difficult to discuss these issues candidly, consider it a red flag . . . What's troublesome now is likely to become more troublesome later.

I avoided the packet like the plague. I didn't fill out the sheet entitled "Determining Your Net Worth" because I didn't have one and didn't need a sheet to tell me that. Nor did I fill out the "Determining Your Cash Flow" sheet because I didn't want to know the reality of how much was actually going out. And I hated the "Your Future Financial Security Will Not Come by Chance" sheet that told me I had to ask myself these questions:

> How much are you saving now?

> NOTHING.

> If you continue to save as you have in the past, how much money will you have in ten years?

> NOTHING.

> Are you satisfied with your current saving plan?

> *Oh yes, more than satisfied with it! I'm saving nothing and can't imagine even making enough to have anything to save.*

> Will I save systematically to reach my financial goals?

For me the question was: Will I earn? not, Will I save? These sheets were not for me. Me, an artist. Me, a young entrepreneur who hadn't had enough time yet to test her mettle. I was totally worn-out by the time I got to the sheet on "The Power of Compounding Consistency." Was there going to be a class entitled "Financial Planning for Artists Whose Career of Choice Is the Equivalent of Legalized Gambling and Who Thinks She's Too Good to Waitress and Temp?"

Long before I had gotten engaged, I told the Notorious DLB that I couldn't seriously think about marriage until I was independent—meaning no longer dependent on my parents for money. Needless to say, I got engaged without being independent, still relying on money from my parents, with John paying more than his fair share. Just where I didn't want to be. Just where I was.

DLB had recently asked me if I thought John resented me for any reason I could think of. I had thought about it and told her I couldn't come up with anything. But after that CPA class, I knew what the answer to her question was. John resented me for spending his TV-show money when there I was, a spoiled brat who didn't give a shit about how hard it had been for him to finally earn that money. He probably thought that I thought nothing of squandering it away. Which wasn't true, but I could see the point that he wasn't making.

So I went to DLB's to report my John-resents-me-spending-his-money-and-probably-fears-that-I'll-drain-his-entire-bank-account theory. DLB told me that people don't want to have sex with people they resent even if they aren't entirely conscious of their resentment. John could love me a great deal but subconsciously resent me and therefore find himself uninterested in being intimate with me. Now that I'd figured this out, there was something concrete I could do about it. I could go out and get myself a good old-fashioned job! Even though I was busy being a mini-Martha Stewart planning the perfect magazine-worthy wedding, making a single Celebration Booklet and designing my sister's friend's condo, I could still get a real steady-paycheck kind of jay-oh-bee. It wouldn't hurt that I'd be out of the house more often. I was hoping it would make John miss me more.

I dreaded what I had to do—some combination of looking in the paper, looking online, calling/e-mailing friends, and admitting that I was a jobless loser who was looking for work. I sank into an I-have-to-grow-up-and-be-an-adult depression.

forty-eight

making money

I managed to suck up my pride and get a job working for a phony control freak who owned a quaint stationery shop in the center of one of the most expensive areas of Los Angeles for the lowest hourly wage I'd made in six years. My boss would soon discover that while I was very good at laying out the text for invitations to baby showers, I sucked at wrapping the little waste-of-money tchotchke gifts using as little paper and tape as possible. And I was always burning myself with the hot glue gun that adhered the fake purple flowers to the boxes for that extra-special touch people apparently flocked to the store for. (It was their signature, she explained.)

The phony control freak made an easy job tough. When I was assisting customers with invitations, she commented that I either gave them too many options or too few. I was spending too much time with them or too little. Fortunately, I was only working three days a week.

At first, I was just happy to have some steady money coming in and a reason to get out of the house. And I justified having such a no-college-education-needed job by telling everyone that the phony control freak was letting me promote my Celebration Books by having some samples in a display window. And I was hoping to be able to tolerate the job long enough to order the super-chic wedding invites I coveted at 40 percent off.

Meanwhile my good work on my sister's friend's apartment led to another interior-design job. I was proud and thrilled to find myself spending my weekends shopping with a bachelor for fifty dollars an hour. And even better, John had just landed a part on an ABC sketch-comedy show, which was a real confidence booster. Maybe with the increase of cash and outside activity, our sex life would improve.

forty-nine

being a bride-to-be

I used a free ticket to fly to New York to shop for a wedding dress—as if there were no viable options in L.A. After days of no luck at haughty, overpriced bridal salons uptown, I found my gown in a Japanese designer's third-floor walk-up studio in Tribeca. I fell in love with it and moved on to shopping for the perfect silver heels.

On my last night, I went out for dinner with my two girlfriends, both of whom had to be up early the next morning for their real, professional job jobs. While we were eating, my first-kiss-friend Derek, who'd recently moved to New York, called my cell to say he might join us after dinner for a drink. He called back to ask if I'd mind if he brought Evan (the Eternally Suffering Collapsible Beauty Boy), who was staying with him for a couple of nights. I hated to admit it to myself, but I still got a little thrill inside at the mention of his name.

Soon Derek and Evan were hugging and cheek-kissing my girlfriends and me. I congratulated Evan on his new TV show. Wishing I was remotely as successful as he was, I reminded myself AGAIN (just as I'd often remind John when he was feeling down-and-out about his career) that comparing myself to others was a total waste of time. *We're all on different paths and careers go up and down and I came to writing late and I can't rush it* . . . I cut myself off. I was too boring.

Soon the girls had to go home and I decided to join Derek and Evan, who wanted to go out for a drink. After doing our time in a too-hip West Village bar, Derek was tired and went home, too. Evan and I, however, weren't quite ready to call it a night and found a more suitable dive for our final drink—or two.

Images of us going back to my parents' apartment and fucking flashed in my head as we talked about marriage.

"So I just don't understand this marriage thing," he said. "I mean the only reason I can see to marry someone is so they don't fuck someone else when you leave town. And I don't think that's reason enough. I love my girlfriend, but I don't want to marry her."

Not really sure why myself, I launched into my version of Harville's theory and did my best to sound confident in my philosophy and decision, which wasn't so easy to do seeing that I was drunk and dying to kiss the guy who had broken my heart. "Well, I think marriage is formalizing a commitment. And if you don't have a true commitment, I don't think you can really find peace in your relationship or real happiness in life, for that matter. And that takes a while—to say the least. So if you're married, you know the other person isn't going anywhere. You have the while, and so you can stop worrying about if this fight or that fight is going to lead to the breakup and get on with things. I mean, of course, John and I have problems. But thanks to an old beau who got me into therapy that changed my life, I later found couples therapy, which really changed my life." I was happy to have the opportunity to thank him. "We're doing sooo much better now than we used to and . . ."

I wonder how convincing I sounded with my knee touching his.

Around four in the morning, we left the bar and had to go in opposite directions. All liquored-up, I ached to kiss him but begged myself not to let that desire leak out of me, lest Evan think I wasn't madly in love with John despite our problems, which I actually was. My love for John didn't stop me from feeling the feelings I was feeling toward Evan, but fortunately it did stop me from both disrespecting John and embarrassing myself by attempting to prolong our embrace goodnight or anything like that. I jumped in a cab and was grateful that the driver was whizzing my desire away from a place where it could get me in trouble.

When I returned to L.A., I quit my stationery store job—the woman was just too hard to take for only thirteen dollars an hour. John was surprisingly supportive. He hadn't thought I'd last, but certainly appreciated the effort.

fifty

the people vs. mini-martha

My response to my fear and loathing of becoming a responsible adult was to become the ultimate Martha Stewart's *Weddings* magazine bride. Becoming a mini-Martha appealed to the aesthete in me, the host in me, the shopper in me, the director in me, the designer in me, as well as the searching-for-a-valid-excuse-to-hide-from-the-real-world in me. I both reveled in and chastised myself for being such a mini-Martha.

In the courtroom of my mind, the People vs. Mini-Martha raged as I worked on the never-ending details of my wedding. I took turns playing the prosecutor, the defendant, the defense attorney, the judge, and each one of the twelve jurors. The charges? Wasting Valuable Time in the First Degree and Reckless Endangerment of One's Finances and Career.

"*The People* v. *Mini-Martha*. All rise, the Honorable Jennifer B. Schlosberg presiding," the bailiff-me announced.

"Be seated," said Judge Schlosberg. "Opening arguments will commence. Ms. Schlosberg?"

"Thank you, Your Honor. Ladies of the Jury, I plan to show you how Jennifer Schlosberg, a bright girl with many talents in the fields of literature, graphic design, public relations, and interior design, to name just a few, who is currently at a crucial post-graduate-school-early-thirties-now-is-the-time-to-get-it-together time in her life, is in the process of wasting almost an entire year and a half of her prime earning and career-building years obsessively working on detail upon detail upon maddening detail of her wedding—the beginning of a marriage which, according to the statistics, will more than likely end in divorce. The People will prove that it is no coincidence the defendant, Jennifer Schlosberg, chose to have such an inordinately long engagement of sixteen months, thus prolonging the arrival of the day she will have to get her act together and take care of herself. Instead of using that substantial period of time to procure a suitable job that would alleviate her parents and her nervous fiancé of an unnecessary financial burden, Ms. Schlosberg has chosen to attack the planning of her wedding as if she were a high-society heiress, which, need I say, she most certainly is not.

"Ms. Schlosberg is taking virtually an entire year of her life and flushing it down the toilet because she is enamored with every idea in Martha Stewart's *Weddings* magazine. Ladies, you have no choice but to find her guilty. This is your opportunity to send a loud and clear message to the women of this society that their wedding obsessions are a total and absolutely extravagant waste of time, energy, and money. We have people starving in the world. Homeless. Wars. Disease. 'Get a life' is the message you have a responsibility to pass on to these wannabe princesses. And I am confident that you will."

Prosecuting-attorney-me sat down. Defense-attorney-me—wearing a much more chic outfit than the prosecuting-attorney-me—stood up and walked over to the jury box.

"Ladies of the Jury, who surely value the most sacred of all feelings, love," the defense-attorney-me began, shaking her head and scoffing with incredulity, "these charges are not only entirely unfounded, they are shocking. We have seen in this decade hundreds of millions of venture-capital money given to start-up dot-com companies only to watch that money be wasted on building companies too quickly and causing outrageous problems in the stock market. And here we have an entrepreneurial, innovative woman—with a relatively nonexistent amount of start-up money contributed by her parents—diversifying her efforts and trying to start three careers at once on a shoestring. And it should be pointed out again that she has already achieved a modicum of success in all three ventures. She has had two interior-design clients. She's been able to raise her rate from thirty-five dollars an hour to fifty. And she has had three clients this year in her first-of-its-kind Celebration Books business. It is true that her profits aren't huge, but she is building these businesses from the ground up. Meanwhile, she is taking advantage of her downtime by planning her wedding. And before I get on to the merits of planning a beautiful wedding, I don't want to just gloss over her literary career. Ms. Schlosberg, through her own quality writing, has secured excellent representation. Additionally, her first art book received attention in both, I repeat both, the *Los Angeles Times Magazine* and the *New York Times Magazine*, and now she has started a new book. Who's to say that a little break to plan her wedding is going to hurt her work? On the contrary, more than likely, the experience will enhance it.

"I do not consider these varied activities wasteful of a life. Nor do I find them to be endangering her finances and career. On the contrary I think in the long run that more than just her family and friends will see the fruits of her labor.

"Furthermore, the fact that an incredibly large number of marriages end in divorce is no reason that Jennifer and John's marriage celebration should be low-key, as if to imply that this probably won't last so let's not go all out. These two people have put a tremendous amount of time, thought, and practice into working through the problems in their relationship, and their wedding, for that reason alone, should be even more of a celebration. I am confident that you will find my client innocent of all the fraudulent charges against her and I apologize to you, the jury, in advance for the valuable time the People insist on wasting." Defense-attorney-me sat down, and prosecution-attorney-me rose.

"Your Honor, at this time the People would like to call our first witness, the defendant, Ms. Jennifer Beth Schlosberg."

"Please raise your right hand," said bailiff-me. "Do you promise to tell the whole truth and nothing but the truth, so help you God?"

"I do."

"Ms. Schlosberg, is it true that you have wasted—excuse me, *spent*—more than twelve hours shopping only for the outfit that you wore to your second engagement party?"

"I don't know. I wasn't clocking in and out."

"Fine, then, is it true that you spent five hundred dollars on a dress for said party and almost four hundred dollars on shoes and almost two hundred dollars on a wrap?"

"Uh, well, my dad gave me two hundred dollars to help me buy the shoes because he thought I should have them, even though they were expensive."

"Is it true you had the dress altered twice?"

"Yes, and I still wasn't happy with how the torso hung. I have since had it altered a third time and now the torso looks great, but now my hips look wider."

"Are you saying that you have ruined

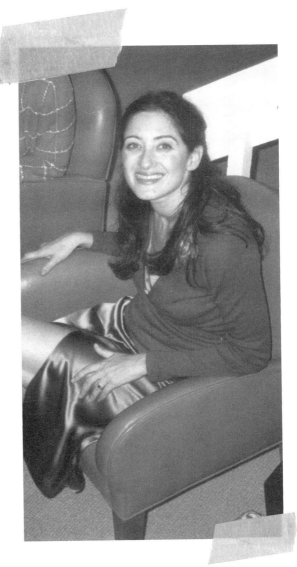

Exhibit D. The gorgeous blue silk dress I wore to my engagement party was being submitted as evidence of my guilt in both Wasting Valuable Time in the First Degree and Frivolous Endangerment of Finances and Career. Shopping for the dress, I never dreamed it would wind up as an exhibit in court.

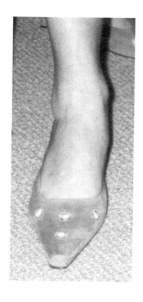

Exhibit E.

the five-hundred-and-twenty-seven-dollar-and-ninety-cent dress?" she said, waving the receipt in a plastic bag.

"No, I'm saying I need to lose some weight to have it look perfect."

"Is it true that you went to at least seven shoe stores in search of the perfect shoes to match this thrice-altered-perhaps-ruined-five-hundred-and-twenty-seven-dollar-and-ninety-cent dress?"

"Yes . . . but the color was impossible to match. It's a steely blue and I thought silver would work and it didn't. I thought thongs for a party in Malibu would work, but I needed height because the back of the dress hangs so long. But at the same time the shoes couldn't be too dressy or—"

"Yes-or-no answers please," interrupted the Judge-me.

"Yes."

Prosecutor-me confidently noted the disgusted look on some of the jurors' faces, women who clearly would never dream of wasting so much money on a pair of shoes, particularly when not financially self-sufficient. Her relentless questioning went on for months and months. The sheer number of exhibits brought into evidence was staggering. Receipts were submitted for every piece of clothing purchased for both engagement parties, for all three wedding showers, for the prenuptial dinner and the wedding and yes, of course, for the bikinis and sundresses for the honeymoon. And that was just for my wardrobe—then came the receipts for invitations, flowers, gift bags for out-of-town guests, presents for our wedding party, and God knows what else.

You could tune in and out of the trial and it would be the same old thing. Over and over and over again. The prosecutor-me had certainly done her homework. It seemed pretty clear that we were losing the trial, and when I'd glance over to where my family was sitting, I'd swear I could see my I-hate-weddings-and-I-hate-being-single older sister gloating.

And still the fucking prosecutor wasn't finished. "Ms. Schlosberg, is it true that in the midst of your panic about having to get a real job because clearly your quote unquote businesses weren't enough to support you, you thought of applying to two artists' colonies as a way of once again escaping your responsibilities to yourself and to your soon-to-be husband?"

My attorney-me looked hard at the defendant-me. *What?* she seemed to be saying to me with her eyes. *How could you possibly have been withholding this information from me?*

"Yes. Yes, I did apply. I'd like some peace and quiet to work on my new book."

"And is it your plan that if you are accepted to one of or ideally both of these colonies for a spring/summer residency, you will go, further postponing getting a paying job, further applying undue pressure on your husband?"

"Well, it's not quite like that . . ." I started to say, wondering why my stupid attorney wasn't objecting.

Would the trial ever end?

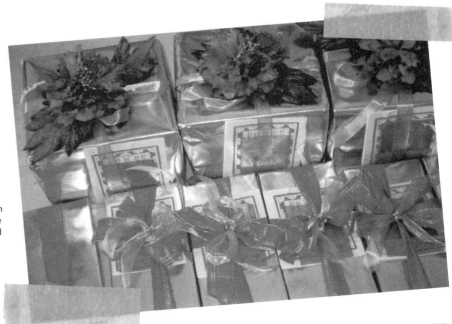

Exhibit F. I couldn't believe the prosecution had gotten hold of the photos of the wrapped gifts for our wedding parties.

fifty-one

one of those

I thought we were really improving in the big-upsets-over-minor-incidents area. I was also starting to understand how things like me leaving the bath mat on the floor in front of the shower actually made John feel like I didn't care about how he liked things, and thus him. Lulled by our progress, I was shocked when I found us in Neutral Patti's office—just five weeks out from the wedding—screaming, crying, and outraged by the fact that the person next to each of us was the person we were supposed to spend the entire rest of our lives with.

Out of nowhere, it seemed that he'd just had it with me and I'd had it with him having it with me. It was no holds barred for a good solid double therapy session. No holds barred like we'd never done before. Apparently not as much anger and fear had been drained out of John as I thought. It turned out that John had secretly been busy adding a lot of ingredients to his Resenting the Fuck Out of Your Loved One Stew—long before he was good and ready to serve it to me right there in N.P.'s office. Here's his recipe:

Your fiancée had a privileged childhood.

Your fiancée is used to her parents bailing her out.

Your fiancée thinks nothing of spending $1,000 on a single outfit.

Your fiancée never had to have a job to survive.

Your fiancée feels comfortable with you paying for her.

Your fiancée doesn't appreciate how hard it is for you to pay for her.

Your fiancée thinks spending $4,000 on a wedding dress is reasonable.

Your fiancée has no savings.

Your fiancée has no job.

Your fiancée hopes to go to an art colony for the summer with no job to come back to.

Your fiancée and her parents just have to have the rehearsal dinner you are paying for at a restaurant that's charging forty-five dollars per person for eighty-five guests, many of whom you don't know or give a shit about.

Your fiancée still can't remember to pick up the bath mat after her shower.

Meanwhile, of course, he was also upset that he wasn't hired back to do that ABC sketch-comedy show despite how inane it was. He was afraid that he'd never make it, that he'd never get the opportunity to get paid to do what he wanted to do, what he was so good at doing.

It all came out in Neutral Patti's office in fits and starts. And I was blown away. He was talking about dinners he'd bought me two years earlier! He'd been mad at me for eating on him for two years!

Instead of understanding that he was afraid that when we were married and my parents' assistance had stopped and I still wasn't making substantial money, he'd have to abandon his dreams of a career in entertainment and take some terrible job to support his new wife's expensive taste, I was so hurt that he didn't love me enough to want to buy me dinner and angry that he was resenting me for something he voluntarily did. It wasn't fair! I was in tears, snot falling out of my nose, yelling things like, "You don't have to ever buy me a goddamned thing again. Please never spend a dime on me. Let's cancel our fucking honeymoon right now. I don't give a shit about going. I'd never be able to enjoy it knowing you were obsessing over how much money we were spending. Fuck the honeymoon, let me use those ten days to job-hunt. I'll start the morning after the wedding; that is, if you still want to fucking marry me."

John didn't feel loved by me because I didn't respect or acknowledge how hard it was for him to spend the money he only just made after a life of not having it easy. I seemed to have no appreciation for how hard he had worked to stay in Hollywood as long as he had to land that one money-earning role and how careful he had to be not to find himself teaching kids who threw stuff at him and broke into his car. He couldn't believe he was letting himself get married to someone who didn't have his best interests at heart. What the hell was he doing? How could he be marrying someone who cared more about her outfits than about his security? What kind of enormous mistake was he making? Why wasn't I just a different kind of person? One with some sense, some self-control, and a job!

As it turned out, every single day that I had "wasted" planning our wedding made John more and more afraid. And with our long engagement, his fear had a lot of days to build. How could I spend so much time and money on escort cards? Addressing invites? Not furthering myself artistically and financially? His anxiety increased with every dime my parents and I were spending. Could it be true that the flowers were more than the price of his car, his new (used) car?! Was this the life I was expecting him to provide for me? How would he be able to give it to me? Would I leave him if he didn't? The more perfect I wanted the wedding, the more panicked he became.

Neutral P. quietly sat there listening to the screaming, the hurling of accusations, the indignation, and the rage. As I cried and tore at my Kleenex, I wondered how Patti could have been so goddamned blind! *Didn't she see this coming? Couldn't she have gotten us to this point sooner? Or better yet, have helped us more so we never had to get this out of control? Or maybe,* I managed to think, *this is just how it works, that no matter how much work we do, it's the quickly approaching lifetime-commitment date that actually brings serious shit to the surface.*

Almost two hours later, we felt mentally and physically obliterated. Good and disgusted about how uncaring the other was, John sat in silence and I hysterically huffed and puffed with snot and tears dripping down my face. Neutral P. looked at the clock and realized it was time to go.

Now? Like this? I thought. *How can we possibly leave in this condition? How are we going to face the next two weeks of our miserable, we're-getting-married-in-a-month lives without resolving this—at least a little bit? Without a plan?*

For the first time in my life of therapy, I left a therapist's office feeling like I was being thrown out. I was still crying, for God sakes. Hard. And it's not that I cared how I looked to the other people waiting for the elevator. I just cared how I was going to/was supposed to proceed with my life. I was furious at Patti and so hurt by John. I was in shock. Fortunately, John and I had taken separate cars. We couldn't wait to get the hell away from each other. As soon as I got in my car, I picked up my cell and called DLB for an emergency appointment. I hated myself for finding myself where I found myself.

Soon I was on DLB's sage sofa, recounting our terrible Neutral Patti session: "John hates me for letting him spend his money on me. For not having had to work as hard as he has. For having had an easier life than he has. For not having a job. For spending so much time, money, and energy on the wedding." I couldn't believe I was marrying a man who not only rarely, if ever, wanted to fuck me but who hated me for letting him buy me dinner.

"What am I supposed to do?" I asked DLB. "Call off the wedding?"

"Well, yes, actually you can call the wedding off. This wouldn't be the first time that's happened. Better now than . . ."

I couldn't believe what she was saying to me. I couldn't believe she actually considered calling off the wedding a valid option for my predicament. How had I fucked my life up so hard as to find myself talking about calling off my imminent wedding in my therapist-of-four-years' office? Had it all just been a huge waste of time and money?

I'd long suspected that DLB thought I shouldn't marry John—though of course she never came right out and said it. I remember, early on in my engagement, when I was wondering if I was doing the right thing, she said I had to "search my soul," that "no one could do it for me." I got the feeling that she was as worried as I was that I would never get the lovemaking or the love-expressed-in-a-way-that-was-meaningful-to-me that I craved. While she did think we'd come a long way, I don't know that she thought we'd come far enough or that we ever would. I doubted she was a fan of the Harville work-it-out-through-commitment theory, although I was too stupid/scared/embarrassed to even ask. I was afraid of being embarrassed about reading a self-help book in front of my therapist! This person deserved the situation in which she now found herself.

Fortunately, DLB came up with something concrete for me to do. She said that before I got married to John, I had to find out if he thought he could truly get over his resentment of my being raised more comfortably than he had been. Would he be able to make peace with the fact that I hadn't had to suffer the way he had? If the answer was no, then we could not get married. There was no hope for a relationship when one person had an underlying, unshakable resentment of the other. It prevented intimacy. Period. Resentment was a relationship killer. DLB said I had to go home and ask him if he thought he'd be able to do that.

I was so beside myself, what with actually hearing the words "calling it off," that I couldn't remember what it was that DLB just said I had to go home and ask John. All I could think about was what calling off the wedding would be like. How I would break it to my parents. How they would break it to their friends. The wasted money. The humiliation.

"What is it I'm supposed to say again?" I asked as if I'd just had a tonsillectomy, my voice robbed by my anguish.

DLB repeated it for me and said I should practice asking it on her. When it was my turn, I couldn't remember the question—again.

DLB offered me a pen and paper so I could take dictation.

John, do you think you'll ever be able to stop resenting me for having had a more comfortable life than you?

I shoved the scrap into my coat pocket and got up to go home, blown away by knowing that I had an entire ride home to think about this shit, furious that I couldn't just wish John in front of me to get this over with, afraid that he wouldn't be home and that it would feel like an eternity before we were seated in the living room, me reading from my cheat sheet.

But he was home and sure, he was willing to talk. The afternoon and space had calmed John down—considerably. He was as anxious as I was to get the fuck out of the have-we-broken-through-a-barrier-or-do-we-need-to-break-up? haze that was torturing us. I reached into my pocket and shakily read him the question.

"Yes," John said. "I'll be able to get over my resentment. I love you—very much. We are going to be okay," he said. We hugged.

Thank God. The wedding was on. Thank God I wasn't going to have to be one of those women who called off her wedding. After all of the therapy, the converting to Judaism, Making Marriage Work, and all of the planning, I'd just kill myself. And then, of course, there would be losing John, the man who had loved me more than anyone ever had, who understood me more than anyone ever did, who didn't shy away from confrontation, from pain, from working, from listening, and from caring.

I couldn't believe the way money could fuck with one's fuck life—and not so indirectly at all. Our sex problems were symptoms of problems relating to money. How had I been so unaware of something that was now sinking in as rather obvious?

fifty-two

the perfect couple

At everyone's place setting at our wedding, I envisioned our very own Celebration Booklet: *The Story of Jennifer & John*. This booklet, however, would be different from the ones my family had come to expect. I wasn't about to write some "ahh, isn't that sweet?" romanticized, airbrushed version of our relationship. I wanted our guests to know that we knew relationships were hard, that we'd worked hard, and that we were committed to continuing to work hard on our relationship. It was, after all, a day celebrating our union and I wanted to give our guests a little taste of what it had taken for us to unite.

"Jennifer, there is that feeling you get when you are at a wedding when you look at the bride and groom and you remember your own wedding," my mother started to say, grasping at straws. "It's so special and I don't think your booklet should detract from these feelings . . ."

My poor, overwhelmed-by-her-daughter's-candor mother was trying to give me yet another reason why what I'd written in our booklet was inappropriate. Apparently she thought it was our job as wedding-givers to supply the ingredients to conjure up warm, fuzzy, nostalgic, romantic feelings in our wedding guests.

"What about the people who aren't married, Mom?" I

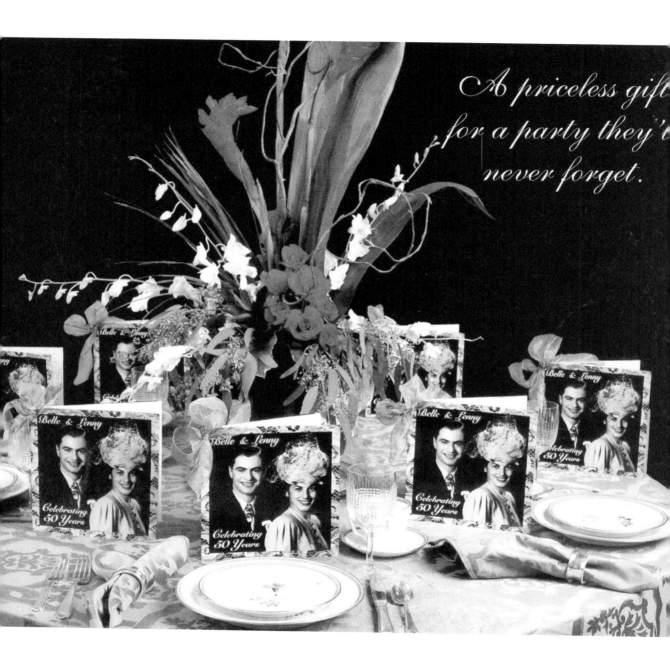

A priceless gift
for a party they'll
never forget.

My Celebration Booklets had always highlighted the high points in a
person or couple's life. And now for my own wedding, I wanted to
document the highs *and* lows. To say it came as a shock to my parents
would be an understatement.

asked. "What about the divorcées and all of their dashed hopes? Or the single people? Why are we responsible to a particular demographic of our wedding guests more than to others? And why is what John and I want to say about *our* relationship at *our* wedding not as important as the feelings you feel responsible for conjuring up for the married people who you think long to remember the joy of their wedding day?"

My mother was frustrated by my logic and my over-analysis of her every word but undeterred. She was desperately determined to make me understand how inappropriate what I'd written for our wedding (that they were paying for, she didn't add) was.

I admit it. I handled the situation poorly. I was a coward. I was afraid of being straightforward. I was trying to put one over on my parents, convincing myself that they'd actually not consider it a big deal. Here they were throwing us an extremely beautiful, big wedding, working so hard to make sure everything was right, overcoming terrible obstacles with the owners of the hotel who lied and lied and lied, and what kind of thanks were they getting? A daughter who was going to embarrass them in front of all of their family and friends by exposing some totally unnecessary/mortifying details of her relationship. Weddings were not the time or the place for that.

This is how a grown-up, mature Jennifer should have handled the situation:

Ring, ring.

"Hello-o," my mom would singsong.

"Oh, hi, Mother. I want to talk to you about something that is very important to me—the booklets for our wedding. I've finished writing and designing them and want you to know that our booklet will not be quite like the others I've done in the past. Usually what I do is write in a fluffy, all-is-perfect style. I say how loved someone is, how romantic their getting-engaged story is . . . you know what I mean, right?"

And then without giving her a second to answer my semi-rhetorical question, I'd continue, "And, well, for our booklet, John and I want to share some of the struggles we've had and how we've dealt with them through couples therapy so that our guests can know how hard we've worked on our relationship and how ready we now feel to make this commitment . . ."

I couldn't imagine me having the nerve to speak so honestly to parents about an uncomfortable subject, but I should have found the courage. I should have given my mother some fair warning. Instead, when she called to ask how my booklet was coming along, I said, "As a matter of fact, I've just finished it and was planning on taking it to the printer today."

"But, honey, it *needs* to be proofread," she implored. She had always helped me proofread my typo-filled projects. She must've started to suspect something was up.

"Okay, I'll fax it over," I said, resigned to letting the storm run its course, not giving her any fair warning as to the content of the booklet. I faxed it and waited in fear. I went to sleep that night feeling like a bad little girl.

The dreaded call came the next morning.

"Hi Jennifer."

"Oh, hi, Mom. Did you read the booklet?"

"Well, yes, both your father and I have read it. That's why I'm calling. And we'd like to discuss it with both you and John. But we'd like to come over and talk about it in person. It is too important to discuss over the phone."

I wanted to die.

My parents arrived at our apartment at nine o'clock that night. As the four of us sat down in the living room, I thought how grateful I was that John was there to help me deal with this "situation." My mother did most of the talking, but my dad did occasionally chime in when he just couldn't take it anymore:

" 'Puked,' " he said, shaking his head in disgust. "You cannot use the word 'puked' in a wedding booklet! It is inappropriate." He seemed to be angry that he even had to explain this to me, *his* daughter.

I quickly scanned the booklet that I had arranged in time-line form.

Puked was under the heading *Their Real First Date*. As a matter of fact, two of-fensive words were under that heading. The second was the word "catch."

> *Trying to kill two birds with one stone—John takes Jennifer to a wrap-party din-ner for a children's TV show he was on. Little kids dressed up like adults play pool and run around. When one **pukes** at her feet, Jennifer is ready to go. They eat at Café Brazil—a charming Caribbean restaurant that Jennifer loves. They talk and talk and talk, get ice cream at 31 Flavors, and end up at a coffeehouse run by high-school students. They go back to John's place and continue to talk until four in the morning. John tells Jennifer that she's a "real **catch**."*

"I can't create a new first date to suit you," I explained. "A little girl did puke. It wasn't pretty then either. But it's sweet that on our first date John took me to a wrap party for a dumb TV show. It shows how conscientious he was trying to be about his career, how he wanted to be asked back on the show for another role even if it was a dumb sci-fi kids' show on cable. And it is also funny," I went on, "that there were these little-kid actors who despite their grown-up attire were really just little kids who puke when they've eaten too much candy."

Well, my parents told us, that is not what they understood from the paragraph I'd written, seemingly attributing the discrepancy to my shoddy writing. Their need to have everything spelled out killed me. They couldn't believe I wasn't a better writer and I couldn't believe they weren't better readers!

"What's the problem with saying that John said I was a real catch?" I asked, explaining that John did in fact use those exact words. "It should be omitted that John knew that I was something special on our first date?"

"Of course it shouldn't be," my mother said. "It would just be better to say that 'he knew you were something special.' "

"But he didn't say that. He said I was a 'real catch' and I liked hearing it," I argued.

Then my mother glanced at my dad as if she was sorry it had to come to this but that was okay, she'd spell it out for us. She took a deep breath. "Jennifer, in our time—and of course, language does change its meaning over time—when one called someone 'a catch' it implied that person was very well-to-do and that perhaps a suitor's motives weren't pure." I guess they thought making sure their friends didn't think John was marrying me for my family's money was important enough to risk insulting the fuck out of John. I didn't tell them that the last reason he was marrying me was because of my fucked-up relationship to money.

Oh, but that was just the tip of the iceberg. The insanity grew exponentially by the minute.

"And how many times do you need to mention therapy?" my mother asked. "We already know about couples therapy . . . is it necessary to mention individual therapy as well? It's like, enough with the therapy."

"Mother, one of the reasons John and I were attracted to each other is that we both were in therapy working on understanding ourselves so we could be in a healthy relationship. Had we not been in therapy, we never would have been open to couples therapy, and had it not been for couples therapy, we'd have broken up long ago."

"Okay, that's great. But I have some cousins and friends from the Midwest who don't understand therapy the way you do—" she tried to explain.

"Wait, are you saying we shouldn't mention it because some guests are ignorant and might think we're actually crazy because we are in therapy? As if the last fifty years haven't happened?" I couldn't believe it.

Then we were onto the issue of "partying." My mother wanted to know why it was necessary to say not once but twice that John "partied hard," a reference made both in the "John Lives in Chicago" section and the "John Moves to Los Angeles" section. "I mean," she said, "we already know he partied hard."

I didn't say, "Mother, John was a raging alcoholic and drug addict who did more than party hard. He often drank an entire bottle of scotch in a sitting. He lived on pharmaceuticals. He did heroin. He drove drunk more than two hundred and fifty nights a year. He dropped acid more times than he'd even begin to know how to count. He was arrested on it, for God's sake, and spent the night in jail hallucinating facing up to five years in prison. And all I wrote was that he partied hard twice and that after he quit smoking 'he was on a roll and stopped drinking.'" Her inability to read between the lines was staggering.

In my defense, John interjected.

"Actually, our wedding booklet is pretty tame compared to the book Jennifer's writing."

I cringed. I dreaded the day when I'd have to deal with telling my parents about the content of my sex book.

"Well, we've never read any of it. We'd love to but Jennifer won't give it to us," my mother said, hurt that her daughter wasn't sharing her work with her.

"And *this* is why, Mother. You'd be appalled."

"Well," my dad said, "this is a wedding, not an art project. What do you think you are going to do with your booklet? Change the world?" I guess my dad didn't realize that he and my mother would not be devoting so much time and energy to making me change the content of the booklets if they didn't think that what I wrote might actually affect people's thinking.

"If I can deromanticize our relationship for at least one person at our wedding so they will not give up on a relationship but will work harder to make it work, then yes, I will feel good," I countered, and then added, "Unfortunately for you, your daughter is an artist with a point of view and I can't just not be who I am because I happen to be getting married. You've spent the last decade attending my art events. I've been blurring the boundaries of art and life for years. In college I threw a party that was a performance! I've used all of my most personal letters in a sculpture! This is who I am."

The night ended with everyone exhausted and anxious. While my parents wanted me to do a rewrite based on their sense of decorum, I didn't think I should just have to guess about what they might deem inappropriate.

Reluctantly, my mother agreed to go home and write down each and every problem she had, and then fax it to me the next day. That was our compromise.

The fax I received from my mother with her extensive problems and suggested revisions stirred a rage in me so deep and powerful that I made a terrible, terrible error—knowing how terrible it was as I was making it but somehow unable to stop myself. I picked up the phone without giving my body the twenty requisite minutes it needed to calm the fuck down and called my mom. I felt so entirely misunderstood, so censored, and so unable to be who I was at thirty-one fucking years old that I'd had it.

Telling my mother I wasn't about to write like some third-rate cheese ball was just the beginning. Whatever disrespectful things I went on to say in my-less-than respectful tone, my dad heard it all, as he'd picked up the receiver without my knowing. And he'd just had it with his ungrateful, spoiled, rude daughter. How dare I speak to my mother that way after all she'd been doing for me—she'd stayed up all night to try to remedy this terrible situation that they shouldn't have had to be put in in the first place. How dare I not care about anyone but myself? He went on to say a few more things that he immediately regretted. What a mess we all were, and it was my fault because I just had to make a statement with my booklets.

I felt bad that I'd upset them so much and instantly became amenable to writing a more "acceptable" version. Which I did with a clenched jaw. Particles of enamel, a result of my incessant grinding, littered my tongue as I plunked away at my keyboard.

Yes, another meeting was called. They still had significant problems with my revised version. John said that now it was time for him to take over. "I'll handle it from here," he assured me. With everyone once again gathered around our living-room coffee table, John told my parents that he'd like to go over every single sentence of the eight-page booklet to discuss in detail any problems they might have. This way, he explained, there would be no more misunderstandings. He figured that this methodical, painful assess-

The cover of my wedding booklet was the only issue that wasn't contentious.

Jennifer & John

January 27, 2001
The Park Plaza
Los Angeles

ment would surely expose the absurdity of it all. *We'll be here for an eternity*, I thought, wishing I could disappear.

"Okay," John said to my parents, "I'll start reading a line from Jennifer's version and then from your version and we'll discuss the two."

About an hour into the process, with several pages still to go, I was so tortured by it all, I said, "Let's just forget it. It's not worth it. I don't want the booklet at the goddamned wedding anymore."

"Honey, we're so close to finishing and you've worked so hard on this. We shouldn't just abandon the project you've been working on for months," John said, calming me down.

I was more in love with him than ever. I was so grateful that John loved me, defended me, and cared for me. I was marrying the right man.

In the end, a compromised version was printed. *This is the last time*, I told myself, *I'll ever let my parents pay for anything because I want to say what I want to say when I think it's appropriate to say it. I'm sorry I'm not the daughter they wish I was, but I'm not.*

fifty-three

tsouris

The morning before our wedding day, the phone rang. It was Grandmother. *How thoughtful of her to call the day before my wedding to say some special words to me*, I might've thought if I had time to think.

"Jennifer?"

"Yes, Grandmother?"

"I'm calling to tell you I will not be giving a speech at your wedding tomorrow."

"You won't?" I said, feeling instantly like I'd done something wrong.

"No, I will not. I'm telling you now so that you can make the proper amendments to the evening's program," she explained, as if she was really calling to be of help, when she really had an entirely different agenda.

"Okay," I said, totally thrown. "I'll tell our toastmaster." I tried to remain calm as I shuffled through the past few days to pinpoint how or when I had offended Grandmother. I knew this call was a punishment. She loved to give speeches. If she was willing to deny herself the rare opportunity to perform for such a big crowd, I really must have done something wrong.

I hung up in shock and immediately told John what had just happened.

"Why? Why is she doing this to us?" he wanted to

know. John wanted the phone. Thank God. I was relieved that I had a stand-up guy to do what I was obviously incapable of.

"Hi, Honey," he said. "It's John."

"Yes, hello, John," she replied, using a tone she'd never used with him before.

"Honey, Jennifer said that you won't be making a speech at our wedding tomorrow night—"

"Yes, that's right. I will not," she said, cutting him off.

"Well, we'd like to know if there is something we have done to upset you."

Not acknowledging his straightforward question, Grandmother only reiterated what it was that she would not be doing and then she said good-bye. John was incredulous and more upset than I'd ever seen him. Why, he wanted to know, why was she doing this to us the day before our wedding? He couldn't take the not knowing, he couldn't understand having to live with the punishment unaware of the crime, so he called again. "Have we offended you in any way? We're concerned."

She wouldn't be speaking and that was it. Once again, "Good-bye."

His calling twice was an obvious admission of our anxiety. She was even more triumphant.

"Your fucking family. They are driving me fucking crazy . . ." He'd had it. He'd reached his threshold and started to cry. And then he said that I was a part of or fed into this outrageous behavior of theirs. "My family is so much better than your crazy family. They've been nothing but supportive. It was enough already with all of the goddamned meetings over the booklets and all of the people they just have to have at the goddamned rehearsal dinner. And enough with your depressed sister, who hasn't supported you at all through this whole thing. And now your grandma! I'm getting the hell out of here. I'm going to hang out with my family!" No doubt wondering what the hell he was doing marrying into my crazy family, he got dressed and left.

Ten minutes earlier, I had been so looking forward to the rehearsal dinner and wedding. Now I was sick, furious, confused, hurt, and fuming. Grandmother was really winning and I was letting her. Why couldn't she be the loving, doting, supportive grandmother that she usually was and I'd assumed she would be on the day her youngest granddaughter was marrying a kind, smart, caring, talented, funny, ambitious *Jewish* mensch? Or at the very least why couldn't she be a I'm-not-going-to-make-trouble-for-these-two-wonderful-kids-that-I-love-so-much-the-day-before-their-wedding-when-over-sixty-guests-from-around-the-country-are-coming-to-town-and-I'm-sure-they-have-a-million-last-minute-details-to-contend-with Grandmother?

Desperate for some peace of mind, I called my mother. Surely she'd call Grandmother, find out what she was so worked up over, and explain it all away. But she wasn't home! She was getting her hair done. And just then I got the we're-running-late-but-don't-worry call from my girlfriends who were picking me up to go get our hair and nails done, which guaranteed that I'd have some extra time to just sit home alone while a cyclone of feelings swirled inside of me. Finally, the phone rang again. It was the girls, not my mother. I buzzed them in, hugged and kissed them, and told them everything. Thank God they were there. We had to run, we were late.

Sitting in our chairs while the Vietnamese women worked on our feet, Linsey and Kim alternated telling me their weddings-always-cause-family-drama stories in an effort to make me feel better, to tell me how this kind of chaos was normal, to take my mind off of my anxiety. Finally, thank God, I got through on my cell to my mother, who said that she had no idea what was upsetting Grandmother, that this was all new to her, but she'd do her best to find out. I tried to make sure my mom understood how much Grandmother had upset not only me but John and how upset I was that Grandmother had done this to him right before his wedding. I needed her to call me as soon as she found anything out. My phone never rang, not at the nail place, in the car, at the hair salon . . . hours and hours of no phone ringing.

After our hair appointments, Linz and Kim dropped me off at home so I could go with John to the synagogue, where we were all—our entire twenty-five-person wedding party—meeting for our rehearsal. John had calmed down and so had I. We hugged and were relieved we had each other. We got in my car and said things like, "Here we go, honey. We're really doing it. We're getting married. Can you believe it? We're really doing it. I love you so much, Angelhead. I love you. This is going to be fun. Fuck Grandmother, this is going to be great."

In addition to our friends, chaos greeted us at the synagogue. The entire block—most of which was taken up by the incredible edifice that was the synagogue's sanctuary—had lost power. The head of maintenance said that it would be too dangerous to have our rehearsal in the temple without any light. The wedding planner suggested we do it outside in the drizzling rain. Not anxious to have my blown-dry hair ruined, I preferred to do it in the dark. People were looking for flashlights. John was trying to weigh our options while greeting his groomsmen, several of whom had flown in from across the country—two of whom he hadn't seen in years. I was busy carrying in the programs, the chuppah, and kissing everyone hello. And in the middle of it all appeared my mother, who said that she had to talk to me and John right away.

My mother wanted us to join her in a corner where we could have a modicum of privacy. "Grandma," she explained, "has been so upset all day that she was actually crying on the phone with me the whole way over here."

Cut to the chase, I thought. "Okay, Mom, what is she so upset about?"

"I'm trying to tell you, Jennifer, just give me a minute."

It was as if my mom didn't notice the chaos swirling up and down the halls just a few feet away.

"Well, it turns out that there are two different reasons your grandma is so upset," she slowly said by way of introduction.

"Okay, Mother, just tell us what it is."

My mother—not happy with her daughter's apparent lack of respect for her eighty-nine-year-old grandmother—took a breath and proceeded. "It's the kiddush cup." Apparently, Grandmother was hurt that I didn't ask her to use her kiddush cup in the ceremony and that instead we were using someone else's.

While this was certainly more than I could take, it was much more than John could. He didn't have time for this pettiness when we had a wedding to rehearse. He didn't have time to hear about a grandmother who was incapable of weighing a lifetime of love and devotion from her granddaughter against some bullshit infraction. John said he was sorry but he had to go, leaving my mother shocked that he could be so insensitive to her poor mother's pain.

"Mother," I said, stupidly bothering to even start explaining myself. "I *did* ask her to use her kiddush cup. I called her expressly for that purpose, with the desire to make her feel honored and a part of everything. She said she'd have to think about it because she didn't want anything to happen to it. She told me that at your wedding she had loaned you and your sister her favorite handkerchiefs but she didn't get them back and she's never forgotten that. So I moved on and got another cup. The last thing I wanted to do on my wedding day was worry about where the hell her kiddush cup was." As curious as I was about what the second terrible offense Grandmother had concocted that warranted a metaphoric slap in the face the day before my wedding, I had to excuse myself.

I found the maintenance guy and told him I'd opened the doors to the sanctuary, that people's eyes would adjust and we thought it was light enough to hold the rehearsal there. John and I took over for our shell-shocked wedding planner and ran the rehearsal in the dark beautifully.

On to the rehearsal dinner, the best party of our lives. The best speech of the evening was, of course, from my groom. I was surprised when he walked up to the microphone with a shopping bag.

"Jennifer is a complex person. I thought the best way to introduce her was through her shoes," he said. One by one he pulled out pairs of shoes:

These are **Jimmy Choo shoes**—the finest-made shoes in Beverly Hills. I love the way Jennifer knows these things. Her appreciation for this kind of stuff is at once hilarious and endearing.

White slippers. These white slippers were meant for her grandmother. They didn't fit, so she started wearing them herself and turned them into a cool, hip, retro look. Next year everyone will be wearing these.

Keds. You can see from the lack of dirt on these shoes that she is someone who enjoys the finer points of leisure. There is some dirt here from Jennifer's one and only camping trip. We proposed to each other that night.

These **hiking boots** represent her method of staying in shape: hiking. But this is a metaphor for Jennifer. Jennifer is strong. Jennifer is not afraid to climb mountains. Jennifer is determined and powerful and a hard worker. She is a tough cookie and a great partner.

Black boots with toes that curl up. We all know her taste is impeccable. This pair of boots, however, represents her one failure. As you can plainly see, the toes curl up and therefore the boots are unwearable. Unfortunately we learned this too late to return them. But Jennifer will be the first to admit her mistakes. She is honest. These boots are for sale.

Flip-flops—mine. Fashion doesn't need to be expensive. These are my flip-flops that Jennifer insisted I wear instead of my Birkenstocks. As soon as I started to wear them, I noticed that every man with any style in L.A. was wearing these. This demonstrates Jennifer's ability to compromise. She knows I have issues with spending money and here she is able to achieve her goal—me looking good—and respecting my money issues simultaneously.

Pointy shoes. These shoes represent her ability to kick some butt. Jennifer gets involved. She is proactive and strong, and as a partner I couldn't ask for anything more.

I knew without question I was marrying a man who understood me—the right man.

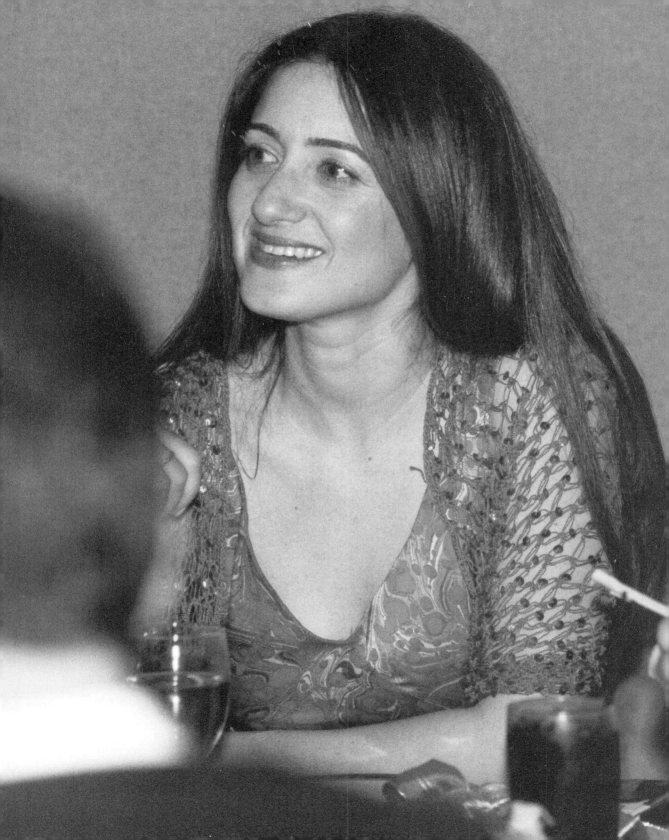

Bedroom slippers. These slippers represent another side of Jennifer. Jennifer loves to cuddle and hold (as she puts it). She is a sweet, loving, warm little love bunny who wears cutie slippers like these.

This is the complex person named Jennifer Schlosberg who I will marry tomorrow. She is stylish, understanding, hardworking, sexy, and lovable.

Despite everything and because of everything, I knew I was marrying the right man. Thank God.

We drove home giddy, overwhelmed by all of the love and our good fortune. I gathered my things, as we thought it would be fun, more dramatic, and very traditional of us to not sleep together the night before our wedding. I kissed John good night and drove over to the hotel to stay with Kim and Linz.

We went to sleep. Tomorrow I was getting married.

fifty-four

the twenty-seventh of january

The morning of the wedding, after the hairdresser's but before I was to be picked up, with my tiara affixed to my head I cleaned out my car to kill time. I gave myself a pep talk. I reminded myself that of course things were bound to go wrong before and during the wedding and that I was to just swing with it because everything was going to work out anyway. I wanted myself to relax and enjoy the day.

And while I'm sure I have no one to blame but myself for my inability to swing with it, my inability to just stop and take a deep breath in and a long slow exhale out so that I wouldn't let insignificant things get to me, I will tell you who I blame anyway: our wedding planner. Her blatant incompetence and lack of common sense sent a low-on-patience bride into more than one minirage-filled state. "Where is the *ketubah*?" she asked while I was getting my makeup done, as if I hadn't shown her exactly where it was the night before. "Where is the chuppah?" she'd come back and ask, as if I hadn't shown her exactly where it was the night before. Her timing was always perfectly wrong and oblivious. *Please, just let her leave me the fuck alone,* I prayed.

Fortunately, I was surrounded by my best friends in the world who were getting dolled up and helping one another with makeup and hair and zippers. Daniel (I had

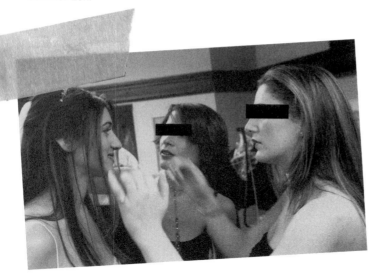

three men in my wedding party) affixed my veil and Linsey smoothed some of my flyaway hairs and I felt cared for. And then it was time for the official portraits.

I walked through the halls of the synagogue with my long veil trailing, feeling very bridal and full of anticipation. I was excited to go see my groom.

I was so grateful to have my friends there to help calm me down—because I needed calming.

To see John on his wedding day with his smile and warmth and unadulterated joy all emanating from his body like heat rising off a football player's head after he's worked his ass off in the freezing cold is to want to marry John. I don't know if the same could be said for his bride. Poor thing, wouldn't it have been nice for him if I, too, were emanating such warmth and love, helping to reassure him that he was doing the right thing by forsaking all others (even though we don't actually hear those words in a Jewish ceremony—perhaps because Jacob didn't have to forsake all others)?

Finally, an eternity or seconds later, I was enveloped by John, who kissed me, loved me, and told me how beautiful I was—successfully calming me down. He instantly knew I'd been having a hard time and didn't judge me or question me, he just loved me, showering me with the hugs and kisses I so desperately needed. It's not like I felt comfortable getting them from my parents, from whom I felt decidedly distant ever since the booklet incident. Certainly I wasn't dying to be loved by my grandparents, not that I could anyway. My always-late aunt would be bringing them an hour late, holding up the service. And it's not like my sister and I had been getting along all year. Ever since I'd embraced getting married like a mini-Martha and didn't show enough empathy for her suffering from the still-single older-sister condition, we'd become estranged. My family as a whole, instead of seeing if I needed anything or if they could help, became afraid of me when I bristled at the wedding planner, and they simply stepped back and out of my way. But John, he wasn't afraid of me. He understood what I needed and he provided it, with a smile and comforting hug. I truly felt like I was doing the right thing. I wondered if the family drama was part of the process of breaking away from your family to start your own. I thought of the biblical passage "Therefore a man leaves his father and his mother and clings to his wife so that they become one flesh." I definitely felt like I was leaving my parents and clinging to John.

Nine hundred (thousand, gagillion) photos later, finally the whole wedding party was gathered in the conference room with Rabbi Schulweiss and Cantor Fox as the *ketubah* and California-marriage-certificate signing were about to begin. And then it got really fun.

But no one could calm me like John.

As soon as our last witness signed the *ketubah*, the rabbi and cantor broke out in song. Everyone was clapping and singing. My grandparents. My parents. John's parents. All of my best friends. All of John's best friends. Our flower girls. Some of my parents' closest friends. Singing and clapping. *"Simon tov vemazel tov vemazel tov veseeman yehay lanu."* Singing soothed me and infused me with the joy I desperately wanted to be infused with. I looked up at John and he looked at me as we sang and smiled, and I said to myself, *This is really happening. Right now. We are getting married.*

Soon everyone in their almost proper order was walking down the aisle and I

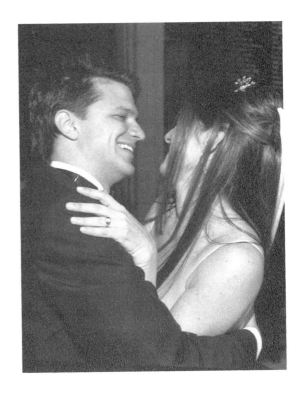

wished I could peek, but I was the bride. Twenty-two people later, the flower girls took off after my sister. And then the musicians took a deep long inhale, followed by the most dramatic cantor in the world opening his mouth to fill the cavernous synagogue with the most heart-wrenching, moving, uplifting singing I'd ever heard as I appeared at the doorway in between my parents. My dad was crying and my mom was beaming, and so was I. Halfway down the very long aisle, I kissed them both as they interlocked arms and went on their way.

I paused and smiled at my guests to the right and to the left. And then slowly, very slowly, I started to walk, but I felt a wobble. So I stopped. I regained my footing and then slowly, very slowly, I walked down the rest of the aisle, looking from side to side, smiling, trying to see who was sitting where, loving every eyes-are-on-me split second of it. On my way to the stairs I turned right and caught my uncle Joe's eye, and he winked. I bent down and gathered my veil in one hand, holding my bouquet of stephanotis in the other. I walked up the steps to the bimah, my groom came and escorted me to the chuppah, and then I circled him three times and then he circled me three times and then together we circled the chuppah as the cantor continued to sing. Our detailed wedding program explained the ritual:

This act is symbolic as Jennifer and John each place the other at the center of their worlds. Seven is considered a spiritual number. The world was created in seven days and, in turn, marriage is a seven-day-a-week act of creation. Our circling symbolically creates a new family, demonstrating that the bride and groom's primary allegiance has shifted from our parents to each other. We are now bound to each other more intimately than to our parents.

After the rabbi welcomed everyone and the cantor dramatically sang the seven blessings, it was time to say our vows. John took the ring from his brother as I handed my bouquet to my sister. He took my hand, held the ring on my finger, and read (from the beautiful vow books I'd made—of course!):

It was really happening.

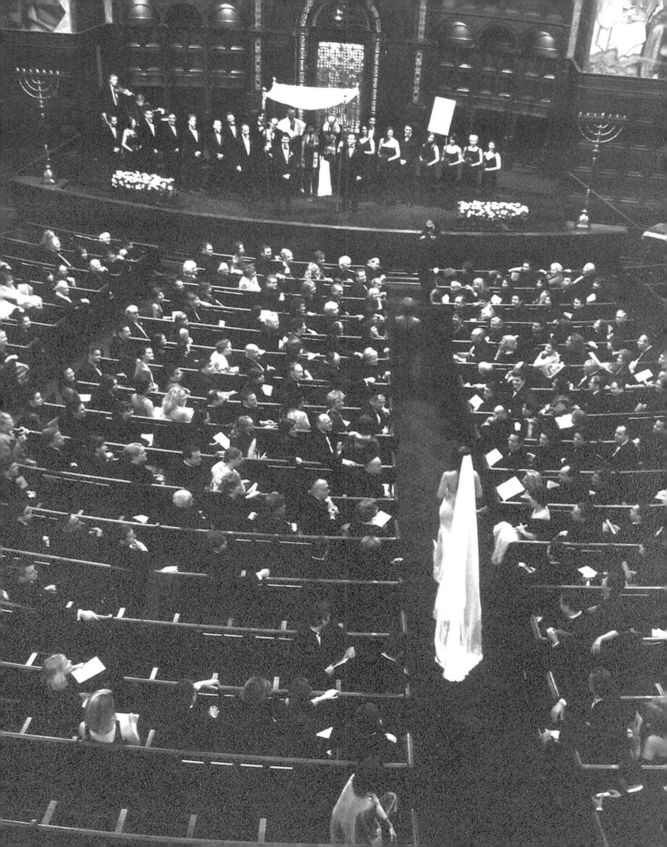

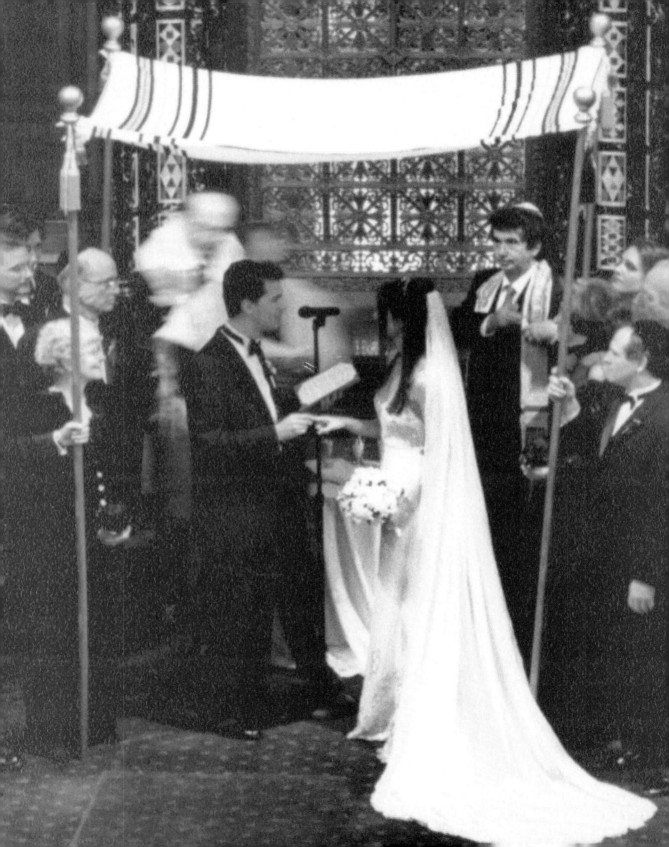

Jennifer—

You care about me so much and you have taught me how to care about myself. I care about you so much and I promise to tenderly care for you the rest of our lives.

I look forward to our relationship growing and changing. I look forward to watching you grow and change. I can't wait to see our potential realized . . . together.

I embrace the unknown with you.

I want to protect you and care for you and cherish you and love you. And I want to be protected by you and cared for by you and cherished by you and loved by you.

Life is more important now. Life is not all about me. That is growing up.

Beloved, you are my goal. You are my priority. You are my life.

Haray at m'kudeshet li b'tabaat zok'dat Moshe v'Yisrael. By this ring you are consecrated to me in accordance with the laws of Moses and Israel.

And then it was my turn.

John—

You are extraordinary. You are brilliant, hardworking, funnier than anyone that I know knows, respectful, vulnerable, authentic, punctual, astute, adventurous, courageous, honest, and you understand me.

I always longed to have a relationship with a man that not only had all of these virtues but with someone willing to really struggle through the inevitable problems that arise when two people come together, in order to grow and to love more deeply. In this fantasy of mine, the notion of what this process would be like was vague, virtually unimaginable.

After three years with you, a man who continually faces every challenge in front of him—personally and professionally—I have learned more about me, about you, about us, and about life. Not despite the obstacles we've faced, but because of them, I feel safe with you and loved and cared for deeply.

The moment of truth.

Haray at m'kudeshet li b'tabaat zok'dat Moshe v'Yisrael. *By this ring you are consecrated to me in accordance with the laws of Moses and Israel.*

Then Rabbi Schulweiss had a few profound things to say. He said that human beings are created in an interesting way. He said that I could see John, but John couldn't see himself, and that John could see me, but I couldn't see myself. We were, in fact, each other's mirror. As he explained that being in a relationship gave a person a way to see oneself, I knew Harville would agree.

Cantor Fox handed each of us an empty kiddush cup that he filled (with grape juice). Thank goodness the whole Grandmother-kiddush-cup drama didn't surface in my mind as the rabbi asked us each to pour some "wine" from our cups into the third cup he was holding. He explained that the empty vessel that was now filled with each of our wines was a symbol for us. It was impossible to distinguish where my wine ended and his began. We are one.

John stepped on the glass as mazel tovs gave way to the Jews in the house singing "*Simon tov vemazel tov*" led by the cantor. John and I embraced deeply and kissed each other long and hard. We left the bimah and walked down the aisle, smiles bursting off ours faces. The photographer captured an ecstatic expression that I didn't know I was capable of making.

We virtually ran to the elevator and up to our room for the *yichud*, where we were sequestered alone for the first twenty minutes of being wife and husband. We ate sushi to "nourish our relationship," but I was so excited that I couldn't eat more than a bite. I put on my gloves, my mink wrap, and took my veil out of my hair while John dipped his California roll into the soy sauce that I was afraid would get on my gown.

"That was amazing, honey, wasn't it?" I said, almost out of breath.

"It was," he said.

"I love you."

"I love you, baby."

We were so happy, our faces made faces we didn't know we were capable of making.

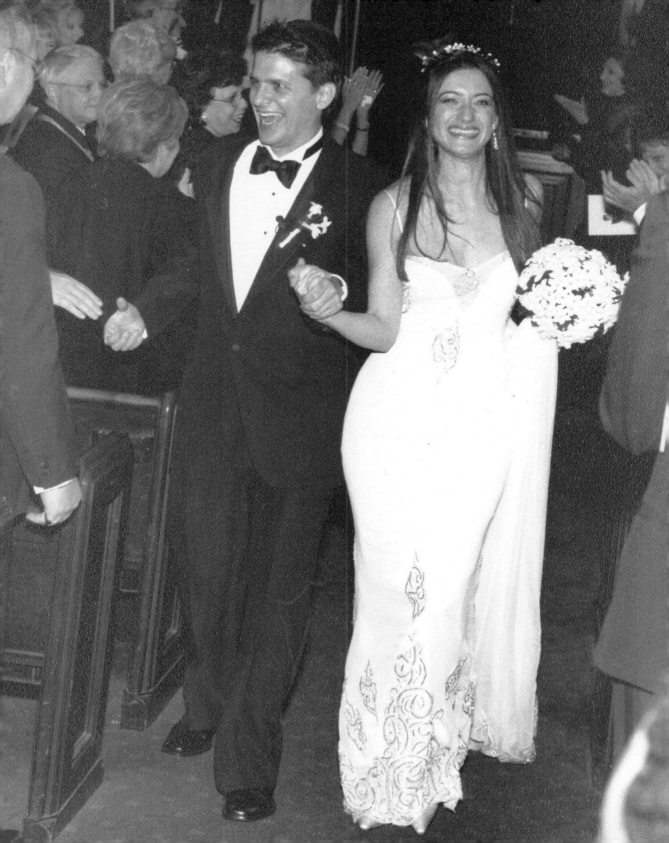

The celebration was perfect, more than we could ask for. The hora went on and on. The room looked exquisite. The band was great—old-school and great. My parents' speeches were thoughtful and loving. And no surprise to anyone, Grandmother had something to say—for a good solid twenty-five minutes or so. She brought down the house. Her comic timing was perfect. She was on fire and she ate up her standing ovation.

It was a perfect night. We greeted, we hugged, we thanked, we danced, we even had a little after-party at our suite in the Chateau Marmont. We went to bed around two in the morning with sex as the last thing on our exhausted minds. Four hours later, we woke up to our wake-up call. Paradise was calling.

fifty-five

paradise

Groggy, giddy, hungry, and good-trooper-like, we checked in at the gate. Only one hour until our honeymoon officially began, which also meant only an hour until the roughly 240 honeymoon hours were over and I had no choice but to somehow morph into a no-shopping, three-thousand-dollar-net-a-month earning person. Actually, I extended the 240 hours by adding roughly another 1,224 hours because that's how long it would be until I'd find out if I'd been accepted into the artist's colonies I had applied to, hoping I'd get to go to work on my book. At least these first 240 hours were entirely guilt-free—I could enjoy myself without feeling like I should be job hunting and eating every meal at home. Paradise in paradise. I was more than ready.

We went to an airport restaurant and pigged out on hot dogs, chips, and cookies—even though it was only seven in the morning. And then, for some reason, John and I went to the gift shop together. Usually, when we travel, one of us sits at the gate and watches our carry-ons while the other goes to buy stuff. Then we switch.

So there we were in the gift shop, him getting Tylenol and a toothbrush, me picking out my usual I'm-getting-on-an-airplane small bundle of magazines. Perhaps this bundle was bigger than my usual three or four, perhaps this time I got five, maybe even six, because after all, I'd be sitting on the beach for ten days and would need a break from my serious and not-so-serious fiction. I went to the counter with my bundle and grabbed some gum and candy. Somehow, between the two of us, the total was more than fifty dollars. Immediately I could tell John had feelings about the quantity of magazines I wanted. Maybe he made a face, maybe he even said, "Wow," in response to the total and then he pulled out his wallet. I offered to pay, but he couldn't stand the idea of me racking up one more cent of credit-card debt. That was it, just a small purchase that provoked some mild anxiety that would probably be virtually undetectable to an untrained eye.

Five hours later we were glamorously deplaning in Cancún, basking in Mexico's balmy weather, taking in the jungle view and the starting-to-set sun before going down the stairs onto the tarmac. Customs, no problem. Car rental, no problem. Finding our way onto the one and only road down the coast, no problem. And then the volcano grumbled.

"Honey," John asked me out of NOWHERE, "where is my toothbrush?"

I was filled with panic. FUCK. Instantly I felt like I had fucked up.

I looked in the backseat and saw that the plastic handle bag holding my magazines had turned over due to my carelessness and perhaps John caught sight of this and had become anxious about his toothbrush falling out. Was it under the seat? Or had it fallen out on the plane, where I equally thoughtlessly stuffed the bag under the seat in front of me, he didn't say but I mind-read. I knew I wasn't supposed to mind-read—but it was a hard habit to break.

It's not like John's anxiety was unfounded. On our last trip together my cell phone fell out of my purse and slid to the back of the plane during the ascent—never to be found again. "Is my toothbrush floating around the floor of the airplane?" my poor doesn't-understand-the-guilty-pleasure-of-junk-magazines husband who had been putting aside money for this honeymoon asked, as if I'd just lost ten thousand dollars.

And being the codependent that I still was, I responded like I *had* fucked up even though I couldn't remember what happened. It is true I was care-less with my magazine handle bag on the plane. But was his toothbrush in my bag in the first place? And fuck, I never should have let him see me buy so many magazines!

FUCK. There I was right back in San Francisco, having left my purse in Steve and Grace's closet in San Jose.

I climbed into the tiny backseat of the car to look under the seats be-cause clearly the yellow toothbrush was no longer living among the maga-zines in the airport gift-shop bag. "I can't find it," I bravely told him, knowing it was the last thing he wanted to hear. For some reason, for as much progress as I had made, I couldn't for the life of me remember any of the therapy, couples-therapy, Al-Anon things I was supposed to do to diffuse the situation. I could only feel my fix-it impulses rising up and my I'm-a-bad-irresponsible-girl feelings quicken the beating of my heart. I was mad at myself for being so irresponsible and mad at him for giving a shit about a fucking toothbrush.

So, as Miss Fix-it, I said the worst thing I could say because it didn't val-idate his feelings: "Let's just buy another toothbrush if we can't find it."

"But what if the stores are closed by the time we get there? Or the town is so small that there is no store with a toothbrush? What if we can't ex-change our money for pesos until tomorrow?" he asked, angry that my solu-tion involved spending even more money.

Still operating in Band-Aid mode, I thought as fast as I could, even though I was fairly certain that we were going to a tourist place, (albeit one that was not very touristy, which was why we were going there). Certainly they had to have a toothbrush we could buy at six o'clock at night even though I couldn't give John the 100 percent guarantee he wanted as if his life would have been ruined by using his finger for one night. I was so frazzled by all of the tension that had abruptly descended on our honeymoon that I wasn't aware of the obvious. This had nothing to do with the toothbrush. It had to do with money—again. Which, as I'd learned in Neutral P.'s office, had to do with trust. *If she truly loved me and cared about my very valid anxiety surrounding money and my career,* John's subconscious was thinking, *then she wouldn't be so selfish as to waste so much money on so many stupid girl magazines. I'm paying for this whole goddamned honeymoon. The least she can do is not go crazy with the spending.*

"I have an idea," I said. "Last time I was in the Yucatán, Pam and I stayed at this hotel that is coming up in maybe twenty minutes and they had this convenience store that has everything under the sun. I'm sure we'll find a toothbrush there."

"But we don't have any pesos."

"I'm fairly certain they have an ATM."

"What if they don't?"

Jesus Christ, give me a motherfucking break, asshole, I didn't say.

I was right. The convenience store was there and it was open and it had a ton of toothbrushes and they did have an ATM and they even took credit cards. We put the toothbrush in our car and decided to eat something at the little rice-and-beans stand. Food dehypoglied John and he was ready to let it go. I wasn't quite so ready, but I tried. I was angry that he had to take away my postwedding high so quickly. We sat in silence.

Unfortunately it wasn't long before the next eruption. As a matter of fact, we didn't even make it a full fifteen minutes down the coast. All of a sudden it hit me: I forgot to tell John that the hotel we were staying at did not accept credit cards. I'd only just found out myself. When I'd made the reservations two months earlier, I'd put it on my credit card, so I just assumed that the whole bill would go to my credit card, but just days before we left, in the middle of the wedding mayhem, I got an e-mail confirmation telling me they only accepted cash at this first place and I forgot to tell John. So I told him.

"Oh my God, what?!" He couldn't believe it. "I don't know if I have enough cash on me to pay for the hotel *and* our meals *and* whatever else it is we're going to do down here. What about the other hotels, do they not take credit cards either?"

"Oh, I'm pretty sure they do. I didn't hear otherwise."

"But are you a hundred percent sure?"

Fuck.

My bank account was empty, so I couldn't get any cash out to help. I felt totally dependent on John. I felt trapped. Usually I would just be like, *Fuck it . . . I'll take care of it, honey.* But I had put myself entirely in his hands and I hated myself for it. What was I thinking, letting myself get married before I was firmly on my own two feet.

"I promise I'll find out tomorrow if the Haciendas takes credit cards. I can't imagine that they don't. They're really high-end places in the middle of nowhere," I explained, trying to get him off my fucking back for a minute.

I could barely stand it. *This is my haven from having to deal with making money? Fuck, let's get this trip over with and go home so I can make my own money so you won't think I'm sucking you dry. I can't take this.* FUUUUUUUUUUUUCK.

We found our little resort. Right there on the side of the road was a little check-in table. Very charming. The place was paradise—huts on the beach, but huts with nice bathrooms and mosquito netting and a hammock. We settled in and I wondered how I was going to enjoy any of it with a husband who constantly monitored my spending. Was I actually reading the magazines he'd spent so much money on? I couldn't take the pressure. *Why did I marry him?* I wondered, afraid of the life I'd have to live as his wife.

We settled in and unpacked, which is when John found his goddamned yellow toothbrush. He was so apologetic. I was furious. I'd done NOTHING wrong. I was sick of being blamed for the idea that I was a fuckup or that I might fuck up not that I *had* fucked up. We didn't manage to fully make up for an entire, painful twenty-four hours. It was most certainly not the way we had wanted to spend our first day as husband and wife.

But we did manage to get over our fight enough to have a great trip. The rest of the honeymoon, as it turned out, was perfect. We couldn't have had a more adventurous, fun, fun-loving time. We went to the Mayan ruins, climbed pyramids, buzzed around the little towns in our minicar, swam in

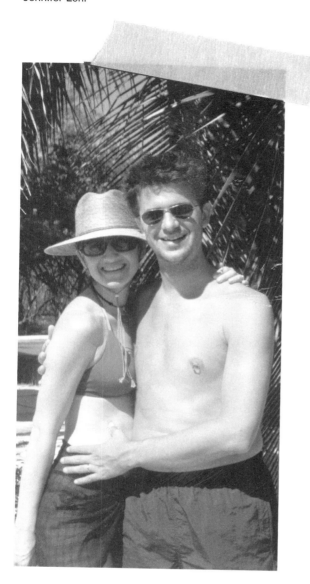

Finally, after a nightmare start to our honeymoon, we became happy honeymooners—albeit ones who were fearful about their future together.

the cenotes (holes in the ground where the water was surprisingly warm and fresh). We ate great food, took beautiful moonlit walks, visited churches, played cards, and loved each other's company so I won't bore you with the wonderful details. And yes, we even did some fucking and sucking and kissing and touching here and there. Meaning three times in ten days, to be exact. And for us, Patti reminded me when we returned, that was a huge improvement.

I still felt like I had to initiate. And I felt like the one time he did initiate, he had to force himself to. That could have been my imagination ENTIRELY. But that is how I felt. I felt like he had to force himself to give me head. But he did do it and I did come. And seeing that we were still stuck smack in the middle of money/resentment/trust/fear/anger issues, I know that whatever sex we did have was a miracle in and of itself.

Days after our return, we were in bed watching TV when we stumbled across a *Real Sex* episode about sex retreats. We stopped to watch ten middle-aged couples—totally nude—sitting on a lawn, listening to the instructions of a man with a white beard. Soon the women were all sitting on their partners' laps with their legs wrapped around their backs, undulating. One came and then another and another, like champagne bottles uncorked in succession. "Honey," I asked, "would you ever want to do a sex weekend or some such embarrassing you'd-never-tell-your-friends thing?"

"Sure, honey."

"Oh, sweetheart," I said, hugging and kissing on him. I was very lucky and I knew it. I had a husband open to taking some kind of Tantric sex class. I wondered if we'd ever do it.

fifty-six

like a good wife

Before we got married, after our blowout session at Neutral Patti's, I had agreed to John's post-nuptial financial plan for an unemployed me. It made sense and was actually very generous. We would use the twenty-five thousand dollars my grandparents had given us for our wedding gift as my salary for the year while I got my businesses up and running. I was to spend no more than three thousand a month and I was to spend it all in cash so I'd know just how I was doing with my budget. Basically, I agreed to become John. I was anxious to appease him and I was sure I could do it. How hard could it be?

A few days after we'd returned to reality, I decided I had to have a pair of clogs. And considering we'd just returned and I hadn't started spending too much of my allocated monthly budget, I bought them. *For God's sake*, I thought, *when was the last time I bought such a cheap pair of shoes*? I smiled at this new frugal, good wife that I was becoming as I slipped them on my feet.

When I walked into the door of our apartment, they were the first thing John noticed and he immediately asked if I'd bought them with cash. And the truth was I hadn't. I didn't have the cash on me and didn't feel like driving to the ATM. I'd already failed and he was already anxious. Here we had a plan that we both agreed to and within minutes I couldn't stick to it. What was he going to do with me? And did I *need* another pair of shoes?

Marriage fucking sucks, I thought. *Now I have to become an evolved material-disavowing monk.* I tried to defend myself. "Honey, I've already made strides. I've put my checkbook on Quicken. I'm keeping track of my spending. I haven't gone all cash, but this is new to me. I'm trying."

The incident landed us back in Neutral Patti's office talking about the same old thing. Neutral P. told an outraged-by-my-behavior John that he'd have to find a way to let it go. N.P. wanted to relieve John of being a money monitor who was constantly wondering if my shirt was new, how much I'd spent on it, if I'd wasted money going out for lunch because I was too lazy to go to the market, if I'd forgotten to move my car on Wednesday for street cleaning and had just blown another thirty-nine dollars on a ticket, or if I'd actually done three things that day to find a job. That wasn't a way to live, N.P. said. He'd be torturing himself and me.

"It is essential for a decent quality of life for both of you that we find a way to relieve you, John, of this constant anxiety you have over every penny Jennifer spends," Neutral P. explained.

John agreed to let me handle my own money the way I wanted. He wouldn't monitor and he wouldn't question. We'd continue to pay our bills separately and he'd continue to never look at my credit-card statements. It wasn't going to be easy for him, but he was going to try. He had no choice really. He could either have a life or not have a life. I was also happy to hear that his psychopharmacologist added Wellbutrin (an antidepressant) to his cocktail and upped his dose of Celexa (an antianxiety).

I was relieved and hopeful.

fifty-seven

one saving stone

The first superthin institution envelope contained what all superthin institution envelopes contain: bad news. From my bank I know a superthin envelope means I've been a bad girl, that I've spent more than I have, that my system of periodic calls for an account balance and then roughly keeping track of every check in my head has backfired. From universities, it is the universal sign for "sorry, you can't go here." So I figured from artists' colonies it must mean the exact same thing. And I was right. McDowell, the famous artists' colony in New Hampshire, had rejected me.

I was okay. I handled it the way I do when I've just spent three hundred dollars on a perfect, yet way too expensive pair of sunglasses only to lose them five weeks later: I flinched with pain and immediately told myself, *There is absolutely nothing to be done about it, so move on. Berating yourself will be of no help*. It wasn't so difficult to do really because I still had hope. I had one more chance, ONE MOTHERFUCKING MORE CHANCE, to escape the pain/fear/torture of job hunting, to escape the bills on my desk, to escape the daunting task of becoming a grown-up—while at the same time getting a chance to do what I supposedly wanted to do more than anything, even though I was so busy shopping for the right dark red velvet ribbons for my wedding programs and choosing the right font for the escort cards and finding the most fat-hiding-yet-seamless hose to hide my fat under my wedding gown that I hadn't done it since I could remember: write. Was I a writer? Could I write? Well, judging by McDowell's superthin envelope, I couldn't. Or at the very least, I couldn't on their premises. Of course I just gave myself the de rigueur how-many-stories-has-everyone-heard-about-a-million-rejections-that-predated-a-Pulitzer speech. I was trying to believe in myself, still holding out hope. Maybe tomorrow's mail would have an acceptance letter from Yaddo.

The next day the not-as-thin-as-the-McDowell envelope from Yaddo came. It didn't register to my quickly beating heart as thicker but did to my excited husband (husband!). I ripped it open and saw the lukewarm words "wait" and "list." Those really were the only two words a shaking-inside-my-body me could take in. Like most articles I read now that I'd become your typical attention-deficit-disordered lazy human being, I skipped the first paragraph frantically searching for the meaning of all the words strung together without actually reading them. I wanted a rejection/acceptance letter with pull quotes. Fuck the cordialness of the *After having read over* 500 *applications* . . . Fuck what it is that you as an institution would like to be able to offer but can't due to limited space, just write YES or NO. SAVED BY THE BELL or FUCKED. One or the other.

"Fuck, honey, I'm wait-listed," I said.

"That's great, honey," John said. "That means you still have a good chance of going."

Having calmed down a bit, I started the letter from the top.

Turns out that those wait-list words I saw in paragraph two were part of a sentence asking me to let them know if I could or couldn't come as soon as possible because they had a lot of people on their waiting list. I was accepted! So in fact my prayers had been answered. John couldn't have been happier for me. I couldn't have been happier for me. I was awarded five and a half weeks. I couldn't believe it and I could.

Before long I was in New York's Penn Station at eight in the morning waiting for my train, carrying almost way too much stuff for one person. After

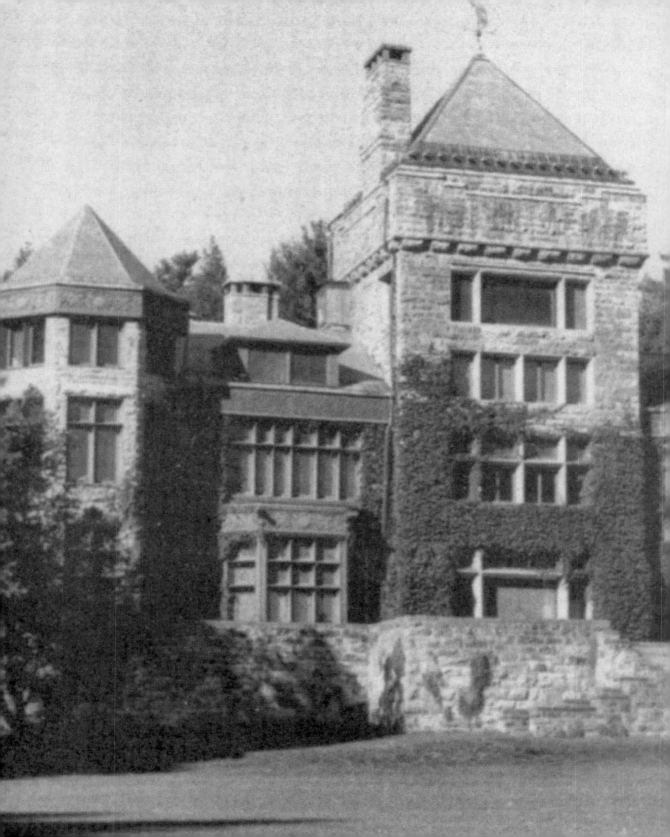

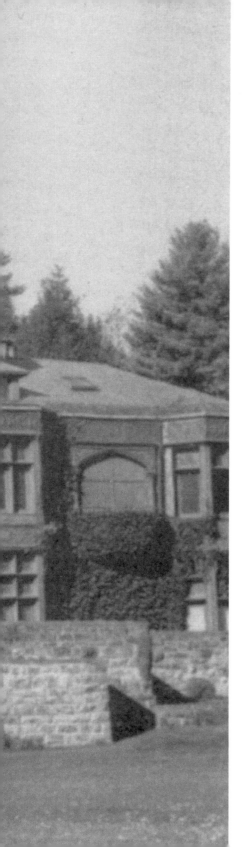

My salvation.

schlepping all of my stuff through the station, down the stairs, and onto the train, I was relieved to finally have my luggage put away. I settled into my seat, put my worn-out, ice blue pashmina over my head, and tucked it under my curled-up legs, used my breath to heat the mini-tepee, and almost instantly fell asleep. Three and half hours later I got off the train in Saratoga Springs surrounded by lots of big trees. I was pretty sure that a few of the other women waiting for cabs were en route to Yaddo as well.

I shared a ride with Caran. A bit nervous/excited/tired, we asked each other the obvious questions. It was so nice to be in a conversation with a woman roughly my age and to be able to answer "Los Angeles . . . nonfiction writer" instead of the now-tired "January twenty-seventh . . . the Park Plaza" or "the Yucatán." Instead of hearing "May twenty-sixth . . . the Beverly Hills Hotel . . . Tahiti," I was happy to hear her answer "Brooklyn . . . filmmaker." Officially out of wedding time and officially in I-might-have-a-real-chance-of-being-a-writer time. The driver turned off the main road and drove us past the ponds and up the winding drive to the imposing gray-stone mansion. It was all very dramatic.

Soon, along with the other new arrivals, I was given a tour of the grounds and was shown my room in what I came to call the minimansion, the stone home where the estate owners had wintered, seeing as it was just too expensive to heat the main four-story mansion just down the path during the cold months. I couldn't believe my salvation was as perfect as it was. What could I possibly have done to deserve this beautiful, this perfect a salvation? Peace, quiet, nice, intelligent, talented people, my own charming Sylvia-Plath-used-to-work-here writing studio in the attic. All of my meals made. A pool. A forest. A rose garden. I didn't recognize myself for a little while—no John, no family, no friends. No dramas. No bills. No TV. No therapy. No couples therapy. I took the afternoon van into town and instinctively found a children's toy store and bought a teddy bear. I knew I needed someone to hold. I always want to hold. Hold, hold, hold.

fifty-eight

light switches

I spent the first few days sound asleep either on the cot in my studio or in my bedroom with the view of the well-manicured lawn. As eager as I was to start writing, I couldn't fight the long naps. My body was desperate for rest.

I loved my life. Everything was better than I could have imagined. Breakfast and dinner were in the formal dining room, where we sat in ornate chairs with gargoyles and Vikings carved out of the high backs looming over our shoulders. Lunches were served in old-fashioned pails with our names on them so we'd be sure to get what we'd requested, whether it was one sandwich or two, or coffee or tea in our thermoses. The only anxiety-provoking rule of the place was that the pails had to be returned to the kitchen before five. It was too much pressure for some, who opted for paper bags that could be thrown out at their leisure. But me, I was always happy to have a reason to take a break from my work.

It took me no time to go from a girl who almost never drank—now that I was part of a semisettled couple who usually fell asleep during the *Order* part of A&E's nightly airing of *Law & Order*—to being someone who LOVED staying up virtually every night until three or four in the morning drinking scotch after scotch, hanging out with

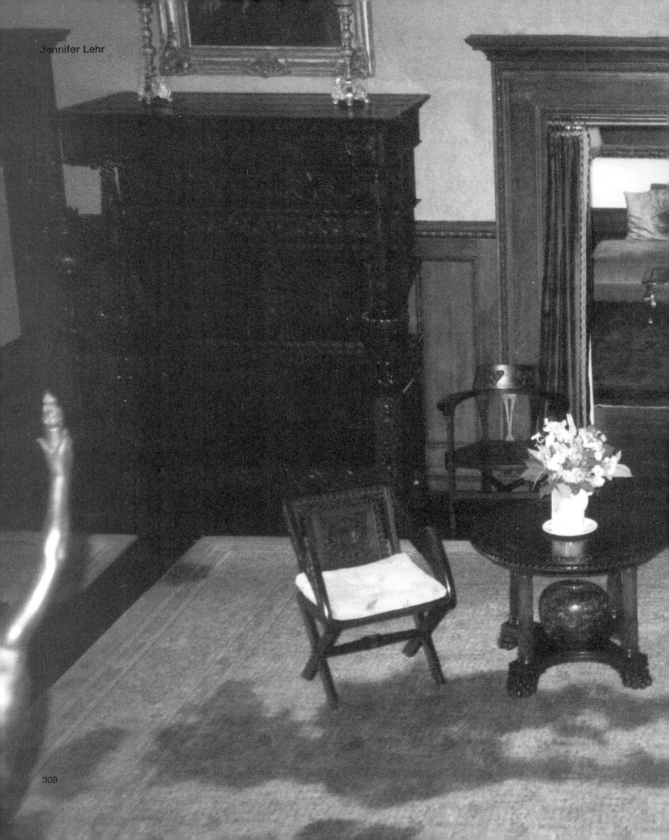

Jennifer Lehr

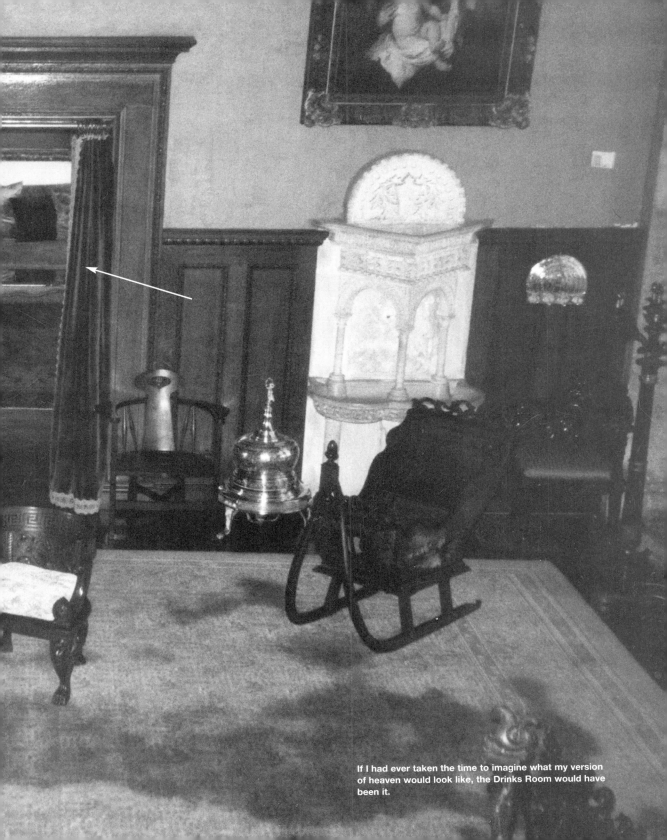

If I had ever taken the time to imagine what my version of heaven would look like, the Drinks Room would have been it.

my interesting new writer and artist friends who seemed to find me fun, funny, and entertaining—smart, even. I almost forgot this person existed. Virtually every night/early morning for the first two or so rainy weeks, I could be found in the Drinks Room. I loved that there was a Drinks Room and I loved the Drinks Room. Dark gold velvet upholstery, deep mahogany furniture, oil paintings hung salon style, marble busts, a grand fireplace, red leather chairs that could be pulled around the card table sitting in the corner, and two heavy sliding doors that kept the noise inside. I was in heaven.

During these first rainy nights, a fairly big group of us hung out talking and drinking and playing a charadeslike game. A smaller group of four usually lingered after the others retired. Two were women. One was slightly older than me and one slightly younger. Both were published writers. Both had book deals. The man was slightly older than all of us and had his first novel coming out the next year. And I—the novice with no book deal or published words to speak of save for a letter to the editor—made four. We stayed up late making friends, talking about writing, where we lived, how we lived, and who we were or weren't sleeping with, dating, or married to.

The slightly-younger-than-me woman had recently and courageously called off her engagement to her alcoholic boyfriend of five years. The other woman proudly told us of an affair she had had the year before at Yaddo with a married man. They had continued to see each other post-Yaddo, she explained, but now were broken up, seeing that he had a wife to divorce and a toddler's heart to break/life to ruin. And then there was the man who had recently broken up with his girlfriend. She was mad as hell and had just left a message on his machine outlining the seven reasons she hated him. And me, well, I, of all things, was married, I felt weird saying. I didn't feel like what I thought a married woman would feel like. But how could I? I'd only had a couple months' practice.

During the relationship-talk part of these late-night Drinks Room conversations, I'm not sure who I thought I was to climb so high up on my soapbox, but climb I did—up up up up up as high as my Jack-and-the-Beanstalk self could go to pontificate about marriage and alcoholics and married men and affairs. I told the still-in-longing-for-her-married-man writer that she should not get back together with him. She said she wasn't planning on it until he left his wife, which he was sure to soon do. She explained that despite what it looked like, he was just this really nice guy who had made a mistake—something about getting married as a way to find stability. It sounded to me like his marriage was courting chaos more than order.

I told her—someone I barely knew—that I didn't think it was so "nice" to have an affair while you were married. I didn't think leaving your wife and young baby to go on a super-romantic trip with another woman was nice either. More selfish and immature than nice. I was trying to explain how being irresponsible and dishonest weren't the likely qualities of a "nice" man. My unforgiving/no-shades-of-gray opinion was actually meant to be cheerleaderlike. The way I saw it, she had already broken up with him and was now in the process of healing even though she actually may have been frozen in hope-holding. But if she was already healing, I wanted to help give her some strength to get over him. I didn't want her to have the opportunity to kiss him again only to find out he still hadn't left his wife or worse yet would never. I didn't want her pain to have to start back at the beginning again.

So that she didn't feel I was judging her, I shared my own experiences about being attracted to unavailable men. From there I led myself to the story of how before I found John to be a gorgeous angel whom I couldn't keep my hands off of, I thought he was a troll whom I didn't want to kiss. I was trying to illustrate the fact how men/women we are attracted to has a lot to do with our imperfect childhoods and that we have to look at that stuff and do something about it or we will be doomed to be attracted to people who aren't healthy for us. (Weeks later, I wasn't surprised to learn that the father of the writer still in love with the married man had had many affairs during his marriage and his wife tolerated it. How could it possibly be a surprise to anyone that she was perpetually trying to seduce men who were involved with other women?)

Despite her experience with her former fiancé, the younger writer still harbored serious romantic notions about love and marriage and was shocked to hear about all the problems John and I had re: sex and money and how we got married anyway. From my perch I waxed on about how for me getting married was an intellectual/leap-of-faith decision, about how I didn't think—leaving out any mention of my major resource, Harville—that John and I could work through our problems until we were committed to each other, and that then it could take years, so why not get started on the commitment part? This seemed to further surprise the Drinks Room group.

Later that night I found myself back in my minimansion-room bed desperately trying to fall asleep but being kept awake by my buzzing, lit-up body. I was caught totally off guard. I couldn't believe that I could possibly have been so oblivious as to miss the superstrong labor-union stadium worker who had snuck into the fuse box inside my body and heaved down on the handle, eliciting that unwritable sound that is made when thirty million gazillion watts of energy are called into action. But as soon as they were on, I knew who the energy source was: the male writer from the Drinks Room group. Shocked by the jolt, I couldn't find the fucking switch. I hadn't even known it existed. I mean, I knew there was that little maybe seventy-five-watt bulb inside me that got turned on around John's friend Movie Star, with whom I still flirted every once in a while, and of course, on the super-rare occasion when I'd see the Eternally Suffering Collapsible Beauty Boy. Those bulbs were one thing, but these klieg lights were overwhelming.

I didn't love it that the next afternoon I found my still-all-lit-up self leaving my studio like a brainwashed Stepford wife, walking over to the mansion and up the red-carpeted drama staircase to the second floor, then planting myself in the proper-looking sitting room directly underneath the energy source's room. No *harm done in just sitting here reading*, I tried to convince my buzzing self, my insides leaping up when I heard feet descending the staircase. Just as I had suspected. The energy source had to leave his room sometime and I was relieved that it was sooner rather than later.

"Hello," I said to the Energy Source, who was surprised to find me reading in the rarely used room. He was happy to see me. I could tell. We hung out a bit and talked. Later that night after the Drinks Room group said good night, just the two of us stayed and talked a lot more.

Trying to fall asleep that night was worse than the night before. There is no way you could be sitting next to me right there in the dark and not notice my body glowing and vibrating. *What is happening to me?* I wondered. *How did this happen? Why do I find this man so attractive? Am I really married? How dare I talk to him all night and lead him on?* I asked/chastised myself. *Now, Jennifer, Miss Holier-than-thou, you are now the unavailable, flirting, leading-him-on one that you learned to avoid so that you could find someone to love.*

Wait, that's a little presumptuous. How do you know he is being led on? Just because you had a few engrossing conversations and because he cleaned your glasses for you at the breakfast table? I shot back in my defense.

I'm not a fucking idiot, thank you very much. He is obviously attracted to me, I told myself, stating what I assumed was the obvious.

Yes, okay, maybe he is attracted to you, but he knows you're married. MARRIED. You are NOT responsible for his feelings. You don't have to not have engrossing conversations with a fellow writer—which is one of the purposes of your visit here—just because you happen to find him attractive and are afraid you are leading him on. And furthermore, even if you are leading him on—which I don't think a few conversations constitutes—you don't have to feel guilty that you aren't kissing him as if you are a teenager afraid of being called a tease. I can't believe that you are actually feeling guilty about making yourself seem attractive even though you are unavailable. You can be an attractive, engrossing person, Jennifer, and not feel guilty about it. It's okay, I said, trying to talk myself down.

Yes, but that's not the problem. The problem is the buzzing and how to turn the buzzing off. How long will I have to lie here tortured by a buzzing body, fighting mothlike feelings of being magnetically drawn to light?

Maybe, Jennifer, maybe you just have to be honest with him, I proposed.

Okay, I'll contemplate this outrageous thought for a minute. What would an honest Jennifer say? I asked myself.

Tell him that you find him attractive and love talking to him but that you are married and you are sorry if you have spent too much time talking to him as if you are interested in kissing him because you aren't, I offered.

No, no, no. I can't assume that he also feels that way, I can only say I feel attracted and am sorry but . . . oh fuck . . . And then, by the grace of God, I fell asleep.

After dinner that next night the Energy Source and I took a walk at dusk down the drama drive, around the ponds, through the rose garden underneath the bright moon, and all I wanted to do was hold hands and make out, but instead I walked with my hands behind my back, each one holding the other from reaching out. After the walk, I went up to my studio and I knew what I had to do.

I lay down on my belly and imagined myself being fucked up the ass by the Energy Source. I hadn't been into that kind of sex since Stuart, but somehow the fantasy came to me. And it was precisely at the moment that I came that the stealthy labor-union worker reentered my body and heaved the switch off because the next time I saw the Energy Source I was surprised slash shocked to find him annoying. His voice was grating, what he said was stupid, how he walked awkward . . . everything about him annoyed me. *Fuuuump*— the lights went off as quickly and as hard as they had gone on. It felt exactly like the time when Stuart came to New York. Someone I was crazy about, on a dime, I was repulsed by. Clearly, my feelings had little to do with the guy himself.

As soon as I was unplugged, I felt guilty as if I were single and we had fucked for real and now I was over him for no valid reason and thank you very much but I never want to ever see you again. I also felt terribly guilty, as if I actually had cheated on John, even though all I did was have a few conversations and a fuck fantasy. What did this all mean? Whatever it means, thank God it's over, and thank God I never had that stupid honest talk with him that would have been HUMILIATING.

But it wasn't over. Soon I found myself all lit up again. It was the rare Yaddo night when the Drinks Room wasn't happening. In search of something to do, I walked up the stairs of the mansion past the area where, just days earlier, I had sat like a puppy underneath the staircase with my klieg lights on, and went to find my new acquaintance Jeremy. I knocked lightly on his door as I twisted the knob and entered to find him in bed, more than half asleep. He managed to mumble that it was okay for me to come in. He'd gone to bed early, not feeling too well.

In Jeremy I saw some Eternally Suffering Collapsible Beauty Boy and thought, *Oh, okay, he has spent his life battling depression and there's nothing I can do to make him feel better even though out of nowhere I feel the need to be his salvation.*

So there he was in bed on his stomach, with his face turned away from me, telling me he had a debilitating headache just like the ESCBB always had. Instinctively, I started to give him a neck massage. The way I saw it was not "Oh my God, I am a married woman alone with a cute/bright/charming guy who I am giving a neck rub to—this could be bad." I wouldn't say that I didn't think I was attracted to Jeremy at all, but the union worker certainly hadn't turned on any lights. I was just looking to hang out and I went to find Jeremy and he happened to be not feeling well and I thought I'd help ease his pain. Too much protesting?

And as I was massaging his neck, Jeremy asked with his voice muffled by the pillow, "Don't you feel weird being married and massaging a man in bed?"

Horror shuddered through me. *How did it come to be that this is what I'm doing? How disrespectful of John this is.*

"You know it would be really easy for us to just start kissing," Jeremy point out.

And then *shuuump*—my klieg lights went on. All of the sudden what seconds earlier seemed so inconceivable now seemed perfectly and frightingly possible and I was again awash in fear of my buzzing body. All of the sudden I wanted him to turn over and pull me toward him. I wanted my mouth on his mouth, open. Desperately groping for a switch, I exclaimed, "I'm married!," to which he said, "Maybe I like kissing married women." Holy shit!

This was more than I could take. He seemed to have no qualms about kissing a married woman, which almost made me feel embarrassed about my quaint qualms.

So that's when I forced myself to stand the fuck up and to walk the fuck over to the divan on the other side of the bed in the alcove part of the rather grand room. I needed to get the hell away from him, but that was the best I could do. I didn't want to leave the room because the excitement generated by the energy made me feel so alive. Lying there on the divan totally turned on, I told myself via telling Jeremy why it was that we couldn't kiss and why I didn't want to—groping for my switch, as it were. I explained to him that if we did kiss I knew exactly how it would play out.

"If we give in to this strong sexual haze, I know that within minutes of kissing, seconds really, I'll be incredibly and painfully turned on, which will cause me to climb on top of you and push my pelvis against your body. And then instantly, uncontrollably, but fairly innocuously, I'll come and then boom the guilt will rush in because I love John very much and I'm married to him and I've just done the worst thing I could do and there you will be, Jeremy, with a fucking hard-on and I'll feel guilty that I'd led you on and turned you on and I'll look down at the little tent made by your erect penis pushing against your boxers and I'll hate myself and my life . . . so see, Jeremy, that's why I don't want to kiss you." And just as I finished my explanation, the lights went off. *Fuump*. I had found the switch! What a relief.

Talking through the scenario was a switch. Masturbation was a switch. I was learning.

The rainy season in upstate New York was over and the heat of the summer had taken its place. The pool was now open and I lived for it. That's where I found a new guest to whom I introduced myself in my I-always-want-to-be-friendly-and-warm-wanting-to-be-liked-by-everyone way. He was quiet and tall and handsome, which his balding did nothing to detract from. It was his slightly hunched back that was covered with too much hair that made me relieved that I didn't find yet another man attractive. I swam, waved good-bye, and went back to my work. But somehow later that night we ended up on the sunporch on the second floor of the mansion talking well into the night. The title of my book was a perfect icebreaker and soon two strangers were discussing, among other things: sexual dysfunction, monogamy, and infidelity. I couldn't fucking believe it. My klieg lights were blazing. Again.

The next day, as if I had no control over my body, I left my studio for a swim because I was hoping a certain fellow swimmer would be there, too. And there he was.

Standing on the diving board in my raspberry string bikini, him wading in the shallow end, I was overcome with feelings of wanting to dive in, swim to his feet, and jump up into his arms. As I thought those bad bad bad girl thoughts, I looked up and found his long arms open wide and I knew that I could not, should not, and would not let them wrap around me. Electricity and water are a dangerous combination. I dove in anyway but forced myself to swim past him, safely hugging the left side of the pool, which is not to say I didn't spend the next three nights engrossed in conversation with him more-than-longing to touch and hold because I did. I didn't touch or hold, save for one hug good night, but I did find myself engrossed in a nightly series of to-be-continued conversations about relationships and sex problems. It turns out that nothing turns me on like a good solid talk about sexual dysfunction and with a real live New York intellectual a good fifteen years my senior.

His room, on the third floor of the mansion, was my new Drinks Room. In it, I learned that for years he'd been on and off in a relationship with a woman who didn't turn him on. He loved her mind more than any other mind he'd ever spent time with and she did have a beautiful thin body, he assured me, it's just that he didn't feel attracted to her. It was extremely painful and confusing for him.

I told him that for the past couple of years, my new husband and I had been having sex problems and that I thought it could be attributed to a cocktail of identifiable things. And though I tossed off the usual list of ingredients, I said money couldn't be overemphasized as a problem inducer, which reminded him of an ex-girlfriend with whom he'd had great sex. She was painfully irresponsible with her finances and ultimately, he admitted, that is what ended the relationship. With her, he explained, the sex came so easily. Her body fit so well with his. He liked how it felt to reach around, curl his arm around her waist, and slide her up and over him. The image was more than I could take. At once I wished John was the type of guy who reached over and hoisted me on top of him and I also wished that this guy was hoisting me, right then and there. He went on to tell me that in contrast to what I was saying, he thought sex should be something that happened naturally. For all of his intellectualism—the books on his desk were way too heavy-duty critical-theory stuff for me—I was surprised he thought this. I was even more surprised he thought it when he told me he'd been in therapy for eighteen years. He explained that he always wanted to believe that with enough therapy anything—even not getting hard when you are in bed with the woman you love more than anyone else in the world—can be fixed, but now he'd come to the conclusion that it couldn't. Sexual attraction and compatibility were not something psychotherapy could fix. They lay in the realm of nature—as they should.

What a cop-out, I thought. Wishful thinking. I mean after eighteen years of therapy he thought sex should just happen naturally? I mean isn't it totally obvious that he has a fear of intimacy if he can't get it up with the woman he loves but he can with a woman whose approach to her financial life irritates the hell out of him?

"Have you two been to couples therapy?" I asked.

"No," he said.

"You should go. You *have* to go," I said.

Parents, marriage, affairs . . . we talked about it all, all night long, every night for the next couple of nights. And then when it was just too clear that we wanted to hold each other and that we wouldn't because I wouldn't, due to my love and commitment to John (even though I was feeling very John-who?) the Intellectual tried his best to seduce me and I was all ears.

He told me that when his parents were first married, his father had had a brief affair which he ultimately confessed to his mother. She didn't divorce him, she simply hung it over his head for the rest of their miserable marriage. Had his father been able to keep his business to himself, the Intellectual explained to me, they (and subsequently he) would have had a different life. Basically what he was saying by way of illustration was that all I had to do was keep my mouth shut and we could lie in bed together without ruining my marriage. By way of putting a cherry on top, he added that when I was ready to do with my body what I wanted and not what social conventions dictated I should, he was there for me.

I wondered about my life—in a panicked sort of way. *Had I done the right thing by getting married? John was the first man I actually fell in love with with whom I had a real relationship. Did I need to marry him, too? Should I have learned a lot about relationships with John and then gone out into the world? How could I have forgotten that the world was full of so much possibility? I could go to Europe. I could live in New York. I could be with this man . . . with that man. Had I ended a part of my life too soon? I only live once, I reminded myself. One time. How did my life get to be where it was? I could have been with someone already successful. Someone who loves to fuck all the time. Someone who objectifies me in the way I want to be objectified. Someone . . . well, the possibilities were endless . . . did you think about that??? Did you? Obviously not!!!* I wondered if I'd made an enormous error by marrying John. After a month away, I struggled to recall what we were like together.

I tried to argue back, *Jennifer, if you married someone quote unquote already successful, you would miss out on the journey, you little wimp. I can't believe I'm hearing this bullshit from you. You have one of the—if not the greatest man in the world and you are panicking because you can't find the switch. You know that you are only feeling such intense attraction for this guy because he is unavailable to you. Keep searching for the switch, you'll find it.*

First I tried the Jeremy switch, telling the Intellectual out loud the disaster that would ensue if we did what we apparently so desperately wanted to do. Unfortunately my speech wasn't the switch. I went back to the minimansion and masturbated to the fantasy of having sex with him. But when I saw him at dinner, I was still all lit up. This guy had his own switch.

My last morning at Yaddo I was sitting in the dining room clutching my bear when I broke into tears over my bowl of cereal. I was mourning the end of my single life. I was mourning the affair I couldn't have. I was mourning the end of my youth. I was mourning the end of my carefree existence. All of my inevitability fender-offers had been spent. I had to go home, face my life, and become an adult. I was so nervous to see John after being away from him for so long. I left Yaddo in the nick of time, unfortunately with my lights still on.

Waiting for my flight, I called John. I told him I was nervous about our reunion—that I didn't remember what he looked like. That I didn't remember what we were like together. That I didn't know how I'd feel after not seeing him for so long.

"Don't worry, honey," he reassured me.

But I worried. I was a wreck—all the way across the country. DID I LOVE MY HUSBAND?

fifty-nine

sexing with my husband

I anxiously waited at the baggage claim for my luggage. I grabbed my way-too-much stuff and made my way out to the curb where my handsome husband was waiting for me with a big smile.

"What are we like together?" I asked as I got into the car. "I just don't remember what we're like."

"Don't worry, honey. You'll soon find out. There's no rush."

It took three whole minutes for me to be back loving him, wanting to kiss him and hug him and squeeze his perfect gorgeous ass. *Thank you, God. And thank you for not letting me fuck up my marriage before it even got started,* I thought.

Within minutes of being home we were screwing on the bed.

After a tiny flurry of post-Yaddo sex, we were back not doing it for a while and I started to feel old feelings and old fears again.

It was the same merry-go-round that we couldn't seem to jump off of. John knew I wanted to have sex and that knowledge made him want to have it less. As each sexless day would pass, I would become more annoyed with little things he did or didn't do. And sometimes I'd find myself thinking about my Intellectual. I found that my patience level had dropped. I'd get angry more quickly. I'd find things John said stupid.

Totally aware of what was happening, John knew very well why I was acting the way I was and it pissed him off.

"Why is it so fucking easy for you to just throw out all of the wonderful things I've done for you and how great of a man I've been to you just because we haven't had sex in three weeks or four or whatever. It's like you are always pushing the restart button on our relationship. You being pissed at me for not fucking you doesn't make me want to fuck you any quicker."

During one of these days, I e-mailed a writer friend of John's who had gone to Yaddo a month after I left. Knowing he'd just returned home, I asked him how his visit had gone. His detail-less response admitted to a fun affair toward the end of his stay. I immediately went and asked John if he knew about it.

"You mean with the married woman?" John asked nonchalantly from the bed, barely glancing up from his laptop.

His friend's e-mail to me had omitted that scandalous bit of information. "Well, what do *you* think of him doing that?" I wanted to know.

Frankly it seemed like John didn't give a shit. And somewhat understandably so. His friend's love life was a mess. He'd string along women he had no intention of committing to. He'd lie when breaking a date or sometimes never return a woman's phone call. And now he had fucked a married woman. He didn't even register for John as someone to judge anything by and who was John to judge anyway? He wasn't into judging. But I wanted him to give a shit, because I wanted him to give a shit about the fact that I was attracted to men at Yaddo and had to try hard not to have an affair. Because it was, I thought, indicative of some problems we still had despite all our work and those problems had to be addressed because I didn't want to be plagued by crushes for the rest of my life. Or *is that just what life is like?* I wondered. Afraid to directly address the subject, I simply but nonetheless-trying-to-elicit-a-response said, "Oh really, I didn't know she was married. But I'm not sur-prised. Something like that can happen so easily there."

That perked him up. "Did you have an affair there?" he asked, seemingly unflustered, though a tinge of panic registered on my radar.

"No, but I could have," I said, not telling him something new but taking a new opportunity to reintroduce the topic.

"Well, that's good," he said, relieved by the confirmation, getting back to his work. And that was it. I turned around and went back down to my office.

My husband wanted me to know that he knew that I wasn't thrilled with our sex life and that he'd heard what I'd said about my time at Yaddo. To show me that he wasn't ignoring the situation, he'd periodically say things like, "We've got to fuck soon, honey," or, "I can't wait until Palm Springs," in-timating that we'd do it on our minitrip to the desert for a wedding that up-coming weekend.

As we put our stuff in the car and were about to leave, John said he had to run back upstairs, that he'd forgotten something.

"What?" I asked.

"Condoms," he said. "Can't forget the condoms."

We arrived at the hotel a couple of hours before the wedding. We shared our disgust at the website's misrepresentation of the hotel and then I took off my clothes and got in bed. John followed maybe thirty seconds later and sidled up to me. *It's going to happen now*, I thought, wondering how it would go.

Spooning me, John sighed how tired he was as my body tensed up.

You are fucking kidding, I thought, not turning toward him, not betraying any of my disappointment and anger.

He then laid out his vision of our plans.

"Let's nap for an hour, get up and get ourselves ready for the wedding, go to the wedding, come home, go to sleep, wake up, screw, get some breakfast, and then be on our way back home in time to rest for an hour or so before we have to re–suit up for a stop at the Steinbergs' baby shower en route to Stacy's wedding."

With my back turned to him, my face half buried in a pillow, I simmered—but I didn't move. *We're not fucking until tomorrow*?! *Is he fucking kidding me*?

I was too angry and felt too deserving to think about the paralyzing pressure our plans to screw must have put on his libido. But then the miraculous happened, I started to talk myself down. *Jennifer, do not say a word. Do not express disappointment. Pretend you are tired. Pretend you are wanting to nap as much as he is. Do not let any unhappy feelings leak out of that body of yours. They will get you nowhere.*

"Honey?" he said.

"Yeah?"

Is everything okay?" he asked, trying to gauge how I was taking the no-sex-until-tomorrow-morning announcement.

"Yeah, honey, I'm just resting," I mustered the strength to mutter, my voice still muffled by the pillow.

"Are you sure?"

"Yeah. I'm tired," I again forced myself to say.

And then moments later, I felt his hand on my ass—gently grazing right around the bottom of my crack. Frustratingly gently—at first in a too gentle way which quickly became an it's-getting-me-so-wet way. Then I chastised myself for being so controlling as to have wished just moments earlier that he'd touch me more strongly. *See*? I said to myself. *See*? *Why do you want to be squeezed hard when his supergentle touching is making you ache, ache in a way that you haven't ached in a long time*?

He squeezed my ass, stroked it, ran his finger on the inside of my thighs. And I just lay there not moving, not lifting my ass up as I sometimes did to give him easier access to the place that wanted to be touched more than any other. My heart pounded. My vagina throbbed and secreted. And then minutes later, unable to not participate any longer, I arched my back to lift my ass up just a little. He lifted my G-string to the side and put his fin-gertips on my soaking down there. He reached up and then slipped back down and then went back up and glided down. Up and down. Up and down.

What's that? Oh *my!* Now his tongue was down there doing stuff. Wet on wetter. And then I heard him rip open a condom wrapper and moments later he started to push into me as I lifted my cunt up higher and let him put it in and fuck me and fuck me and fuck me with my face still smashed in the mattress as my thoughts were finally obliterated. He had fucked the fuck out of me.

"I thought we weren't fucking until the morning?" I said after my worn-out self caught my breath a bit.

John admitted that after the pressure was off he was able to feel turned on. I was so proud of myself for just lying there, for not being a pressure cooker. I thanked John for the best sex I'd ever had, news he was proud to report to everyone at our table at the wedding.

sixty

becoming carly

Overnight John and I did not morph into a we-love-to-fuck-all-the-time couple. We didn't and we don't. However, over a 2.5-year period we did gradually become a we-like-to-screw-maybe-four-or-five-times-a-month couple. I usually am up for about five and him four, though once properly introduced to the subject by something like having his dick sucked while he watches TV, John is easily up for five. We like to do it in the afternoon. We're usually too tired at night and feel like we have too much to accomplish in the morning. However, I'd be remiss if I didn't tell you that we even did it twice in one afternoon rather recently, an unprecedented event that repeated itself about a month later.

When we screw, I feel like we're sexing it. I feel like I'm sexing someone who is my whole life who I love to be with. I do not feel like I'm "making love" the way I fantasized about what it would be like as a teenager who longed to be made love to by a man who loved me. I can love sexing and I can like sexing and I always absolutely adore John, but sex to me is not love-song music in the background as John gently strokes my face before we move our bodies united in undulating unison.

What John and I do, as far as I'm concerned, is make love to each other all day long. I'm always loving him, kissing him, squeezing him, admiring his nudities, salivating over his ass. And John is no longer overwhelmed by my attention. He's now grateful to be loved by me as much as he is. And he loves to hold me. Certainly not as obsessively as I love to hold him, but definitely enough. We honestly just absolutely to the ends of the earth care about each other. We love each other's company. We respect each other's opinions. We can't wait for the end of the day when we get to drop into bed together. And I, personally, live for the alarm going off every morning so we can go in and out of sleep, readjusting our positions of embracing in every which way.

How did I morph into a woman who feels like she is Carly Simon singing, N*obody does it better. Makes me feel sad for the rest. Nobody does it half as good as you. Baby, you're the best*? You, of course, meaning John.

Did it help that I've been financially successful these past two-plus married years? That both my Celebration Book and interior-design businesses have taken off? That we basically split our expenses though we don't nickel-and-dime each other? That John never ever opens my MasterCard bill? That we've managed to seamlessly integrate "I" messages and the like without needing to think about it? That our greatest concern is how the other feels? That I do everything I can to help John pursue his career? That his series of brilliant one-man shows have been an enormous success? That we lead very busy/interesting lives both separate from each other and together? That Propecia has worked its way through John's system, so it's much easier for him to get turned on? That his consistent AA work has created a spiritual Jedi warrior out of him? That it's given him a faith and the strength to face his fears? That our sexing is not such a heavy occasion? That I'm working on being a better roommate by cleaning the dishes and buying toiletries once in a while? That his antidepressants work? That I know him staring at the TV screen means he doesn't hear what I'm saying and not that he doesn't care what I'm saying? That he knows I'm happy that he's playing Nintendo because it's a relaxing escape from the world and not from me? That we are quick to apologize to each other when we've

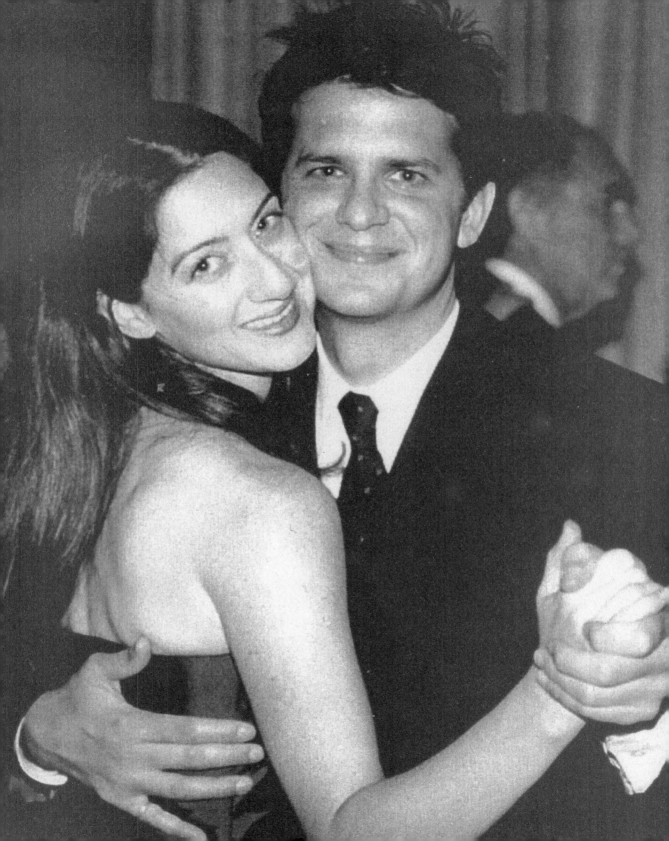

obviously been hurtful? That we tell each other when we're starting to re-sent the other? That hearing the other's resentments isn't a cause for freak-ing out? That he's made some sort of peace with my clothes shopping? That I buy all of John's clothes for him so he never has to know how much it costs for him to look so goddamned cute? That we schedule sex sometimes be-cause we're so busy? That we're okay if we break the appointment? Yes, to everything.

All of those yeses have eroded our fears—our fear of not being what we think the other wants us to be, our fear of not being understood, and most of all our fear of not being truly loved or cared about for who we are. John loves me. He loved 78 *Drawings of My Face*—when others shunned me. He defended my wedding booklet—when my parents objected. And he kept on doing everything he could when our relationship looked bleak. Nothing is better than being loved for who you are.

Which is not to say we don't worry about our careers. We do. We wonder if we'll make enough money to buy a house we like and we wonder if we want to have kids. But we fear those things together. But in terms of this story, I, Miss I-hate-Hollywood-romantic-comedies-with-their-faux-happy-endings have to say the ending to this story is decidedly happy—ecstatic even. I'm at peace, I like the work I'm doing, and every day I can't imagine loving John more than I do. But then the next day comes, and I love him more.

Credits roll to Carly belting out, *Nobody does it better, makes me feel sad for the rest. Nobody does it half as good as you. Baby, you're the best.*

Baby, baby, he's the best.

afterword

and now a word from the husband

This woman I used to know left her husband. She went off to some artist colony, met a guy, and ran off with him to Florida. I didn't know what an artist colony was then, but you can bet I remembered this incident when my wife was accepted to Yaddo—the famous artist colony in upstate New York. My friend Noah told me that these artist colonies were sexual free-for-alls. Yes, a lot of writing gets done, but a lot of other stuff gets done there, too. Now, I don't care if you are Stephen King or one of those guys who brags that he writes every episode of his TV show by himself, but my experience is that after four hours of continuous writing, you're done. That leaves twenty hours of sleep and . . . research—if you know what I'm saying.

So when my wife came back from this artist colony and told me some guy turned her on, you'd think I'd panic. I didn't. My wife says a lot of things. On our first date she talked for five hours straight and I fell in love with her. She writes a lot of things, too. As you now know, she wrote a 350-page book about our sex life. Or rather our lack of sex life. Don't you love the photos? Everyone's face is blacked out . . . except mine!

Now, I wasn't always the impotent, fearful, half-man my wife paints me as in this book. No, friend, I used to rock hard. I had shoulder-length hair, an alcohol addiction, and a taste for the pharmaceutical drugs stolen out of your medicine cabinet. I smoked three packs a day, sampled heroin, and once spent the night with two large sisters and their larger friend in a trailer home in a small town in the Ozarks. The word *flaccid* was never used when you referred to me. I was a wham-banger, ladies and gentlemen. A maverick. A nut.

So when my wife tells me she had some tremors of sexual electricity to-ward some geeky writer at some artist colony, I'm saying inside: "Bring it on." I know my wife and I know that she would never cheat on me. Cheating in her world is panicking about some guy she accidentally flirted with in the drinks room of a fancy writer's colony. Drinks room. *Please.* I had sex on the fairway of a golf course in Edinburgh, Scotland, for crying out loud. I spent the night on acid in a county jail. I know a little bit about breaking rules and my wife just doesn't have it in her.

So, John. Tough guy. What happened to you? When did you get flaccid? Was it going sober? Was it the antidepressants you were prescribed when they found out you were clinically depressed and had been self-medicating with alcohol for fifteen years? Was it the Propecia you took like clockwork knowing the one reason your wife actually *would* leave was if you were bald? Sure. But the main reason I lost interest in sex with my wife? It wasn't dan-gerous anymore. I wasn't with the bartender in her room above the bar after hours. I wasn't with the gorgeous Polynesian woman while a party was go-ing on around us. And I certainly wasn't with the transvestite in the back-seat of a car.

Nope. I was sober and married. And let me tell you that this was the scariest place I'd ever been. Here you are with this amazing woman and then things go south and you are in therapy, A.A., and couples' therapy try-ing to figure out why you don't want her physically but at the same time knowing you would die without her.

So when she comes back from Yaddo and tells me she thought about getting it on with this writer, I'm thinking: "Jesus, woman, I got enough going on here. You take this one. You decide whether you sleep with that guy or not. I'm trying to keep my brain from exploding by telling you my feelings without any Percocet and Pabst."

But, right after that freak-out thought, another one came through: "I trust this woman." And I haven't trusted—well, anyone. Not like I trust her. Boys, I recommend the couples' therapy. If you like the wild side, if you like going to that dark place, it's the place to be. I mean how often do you get a chance to be in a room with only two exits? Thankfully, Jennifer and I exited the door marked "stay together," and even if she didn't know it, I knew she wouldn't cheat. I trust her. And, the funny thing is, after I realized I trusted her, I started wanting to have sex with her.

credits

john lehr

Every day I can't believe my good fortune for getting to spend my life with John Lehr, the most brave, supportive, humble, loving man I know. Without his encouragement, belief in my work and willingness to let me share such private stories about our lives, this book would have been entirely impossible. I am truly blessed and grateful.

susan golomb literary agency

By signing me to her literary agency after reading only a partial manuscript, Susan gave me the light at the end of what would be a six-year tunnel. Her consistent support, generous and understanding ear, astute comments and incredibly high standards continue to be invaluable. I also have greatly appreciated Kim Goldstein's perceptive read and unflagging help throughout the process of publication. And finally to Amira Pierce, thank you for your conscientiousness, support, and calming voice.

daniel hernandez

No friend has read Ill-Equipped for a Life of Sex more times than Daniel. From my very first draft of chapter one that never made it anywhere near publication, he's patiently seen the book evolve radically over the years. When I'd inevitably hand him yet another version of the manuscript, he'd accept it with a smile on his face as he thought to himself, "not again." But then he'd go ahead and read it from cover to cover, always returning with invaluable comments and tons of encouragement. He was the book's first champion. Thank you.

joey syracuse
The most compulsively honest person I know, Joey told me that while he loved my writing, my storytelling was weak—at best. Joey's continuous support made me feel not alone in the very lonely process of writing a book. "Have you heard from your agent yet?" he'd ask as if it was his life on the line. Joey is the best coach a friend could ask for.

lisa addario and linsey lebowitz
Smart, thoughtful, caring, and so helpful. All the time. Thank you.

phil pavel
Phil made having explicit conversations about sex and relationships easy. He was always there for me when I needed to test out some material. An early supporter of the project, Phil made sure there was a way for me to work in a more-than-ideal environment while being well-fed without having to deplete my already depleted bank account. Thank you.

marlene adelstein
Marlene's careful reading and thoughtful edits tremendously helped tighten a way too long and rambling manuscript. I'm grateful.

john baldessari
In his own Gentle-Ben way, John saw the writer in me before I did and encouraged me to do something I had no idea I was dying to do. He changed my whole life.